# Maximize Patient Safety with Advanced Root Cause Analysis

From the Partners of Performance Improvement International
**Catherine Corbett, CQM** • **Craig Clapper, PE, CQM** • **Kerry M. Johnson**
with **Richard A. Sheff, MD**

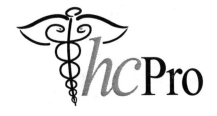

Catherine Corbett, CQM, Author
Craig Clapper, PE, CQM, Author
Kerry M. Johnson, Author
Richard A. Sheff, MD, Author
Charles A. Corbett, Contributor
Ilene G. MacDonald, Managing Editor

Mike Mirabello, Senior Graphic Artist
Matthew Sharpe, Graphic Artist
Michael Michaud, Layout Artist
Steven DeGrappo, Cover Designer
Matthew Cann, Group Publisher
Suzanne Perney, Publisher

Arrangements can be made for quantity discounts. For more information, contact:
HCPro. Inc.
P.O. Box 1168
Marblehead, MA 01945
Telephone: 800/650-6787 or 781/639-1872
Fax: 781/639-2982
E-mail: customerservice@hcpro.com

**Visit HCPro at its World Wide Web sites:**
*www.hcmarketplace.com, www.hcpro.com,* and *www.himinfo.com.*

# Contents

# About the Authors

## Catherine Corbett, CQM

**Catherine Corbett, CQM,** is a partner in Performance Improvement International (PII) with more than 29 years of experience in the nuclear power industry. She has also worked in manufacturing, health care, and government services. She developed and helped implement the first comprehensive human-error prevention program in the nuclear power industry. This program resulted in a complete turn-around in performance for the receiving organizations. Corbett is also a sought-after trainer and speaker.

## Craig Clapper, PE, CQM

**Craig Clapper, PE, CQM,** is the chief operating officer for PII with more than 16 years of experience in nuclear power, transportation, manufacturing, and health care. He specializes in technology-based approaches to preventing human errors and has implemented performance improvement programs for several large organizations.

## Kerry M. Johnson

**Kerry M. Johnson** is a founding and senior partner in PII with more than 20 years of experience in nuclear power, manufacturing, government facilities, and health care. Johnson has conducted hundreds of seminars and training programs on human-error reduction and related topics. He has designed and helped implement human performance improvement programs for several large organizations, many resulting in a reduction of human errors by a factor of eight or more in less than two years.

## Richard A. Sheff, MD

**Richard A. Sheff, MD,** is vice president of consulting and education at The Greeley Company, a division of HCPro, Inc. He provides consulting in several areas, including hospital and medical staff performance improvement, managing poor quality and disruptive physicians, medical staff reengineering, strategic planning, credentialing and privileging, and more. Sheff is a family physician with extensive experience in health care administration and managed care.

# Foreword

You hold in your hands just what you've always wanted: another book on root cause analysis (RCA). Or perhaps you hold this book in your hands wondering why in the world health care might need another book about RCA. After all, health care leaders have been conducting RCAs since 1996. By now we should be pretty good at it.

But are we?

In 1996, the Joint Commission on Accreditation of Healthcare Organizations (JCAHO) established the first standards that addressed sentinel events in the wake of highly publicized tragedies resulting from medical errors. These high-profile cases—the death of a young woman from a chemotherapy drug overdose at Dana Farber Cancer Institute in Boston, the amputation of a patient's wrong leg at University Community Hospital in Tampa, the discharge of a baby to the wrong mother at the University of Virginia Medical Center—stemmed from excellent hospitals that gave high-quality care most of the time. Legislators, accreditors, and the public demanded to know how such errors could have happened, and what should be done to prevent them.

In this high-pressure environment, the JCAHO's standards introduced health care leaders to new terms: sentinel event and RCA. The JCAHO provided a draft definition of a sentinel event, but still required each hospital to come up with its own. Once organizations defined which incidents it considered sentinel events, the JCAHO required them to conduct a "thorough and credible" RCA on each one.

But what did a "thorough and credible" RCA look like? Few—if any—health care leaders knew the answer to this question. The JCAHO provided templates and education to help us get started. We began to learn new tools, such as asking "why" five times and filling out a fish-bone diagram. Then we held our breath, wondering if the RCAs we carried out using these tools would meet JCAHO's criteria for being "thorough and credible."

Unfortunately for health care, they did.

Of course JCAHO's initial goal was to get health care leaders to look at, and learn from, mistakes that happened in our own hospitals. The accreditor was successful in this effort. Next, the JCAHO wanted us to learn from others' mistakes. In 1998 it established a sentinel event database, hoping to help accelerate learning in our field. But fear of discoverability severely undercut the success of this effort. We began to receive JCAHO's *Sentinel Event Alerts*, which are published articles that featured common sentinel events and provided recommendations to prevent them from happening at our own institutions.

While these efforts were under way, we continued to ask "Why?" five times and fill in fish-bone diagrams. And JCAHO surveyors kept accepting our efforts as "thorough and credible."

The Institute of Medicine (IOM) report, *To Err is Human: Building a Safer Health System*, released in November 1999, shook the entire country with the startling statistic that we kill between 44,000 and 98,000 patients a year in America's hospitals. Almost in direct response, July 2001 saw the introduction of JCAHO's new patient safety standards. These were followed in 2003 with annual JCAHO National Patient Safety Goals. Along the way, the IOM released a follow-up report—*Crossing the Quality Chasm*—a scathing critique of our health care system's quality that called for wholesale redesign of how we provide care.

Still, we continued to ask "why" five times and fill in our fish-bone diagrams. And JCAHO surveyors kept accepting our efforts as "thorough and credible."

But they weren't. Compared to other high-risk industries that have conducted RCAs for decades, the RCAs we have come to accept in health care as "thorough and credible" are strikingly rudimentary. At best they have been marginally effective. In addition to JCAHO surveyors accepting our efforts as adequate, three other barriers have kept health care leaders from moving beyond elementary RCAs.

## Barriers to thorough and credible RCA

First, we have not effectively applied the RCA tools handed to us. The best example of this is the fish-bone diagram. We busily draw lines off of lines off of lines, and fill them in with snippets of insight about how we went wrong. The problem is that by the time we've filled in all the lines, we really do not understand how the myriad pieces of insight captured on the page worked together to create a tragedy. In this way the fish-bone is deceptive: It is easy to complete, yet difficult to use. A thoroughly completed fish-bone diagram looks very impressive, but does not necessarily lead us to identify true root causes or to select the best corrective actions.

The second barrier is the RCA tools themselves. Asking "why" five times and also completing a fish-bone diagram can lead to interesting and insightful discussions. But both of these are inherently subjective tools. They entail significant observer bias and variation and are difficult to validate.

The third, and perhaps most challenging barrier, is that health care leaders and managers are drawn to simple solutions. Asking "why" five times and filling in lines on a single page to create a fish-bone diagram are seductively simple tools. Unfortunately, health care has grown so dramatically in complexity that these tools are not adequate for analyzing and changing how we do what we do. Peter Drucker, one of the world's greatest experts in management, describes hospitals as probably the most complex organization ever designed by human beings. Within hospitals, siloed professional groups and departments carry out highly technical and risky activities with extraordinarily complex and rapidly changing technology. The input into this system is perhaps the most complex one could ever imagine: an ill, often fragile human being. That we achieve positive health outcomes from these efforts is a testimony to the dedication, hard work, and skills of everyone working in health care.

But as complexity has grown in health care, our management methods have not. Technology-based RCAs, as described in this book, bring the necessary level of tools and methods health care requires to accurately and effectively learn from our errors and prevent them in the future.

## The PII methodology

In our work with hospitals across the country on sentinel events and medical errors, The Greeley Company came to recognize these limitations. We knew there had to be a better approach. The key came when we looked outside of health care. Other high-risk industries have tackled the problems of human errors and system failures. Industries such as aerospace, aeronautics, manufacturing, and nuclear energy have demonstrated much greater success in reducing errors and improving quality than has health care. Is this because health care truly is different, as so many of us are tempted to claim? Perhaps, but we at The Greeley Company set out to find out what we could learn from other industries outside of health care about improving safety and reducing errors.

When we compared the best approaches to reducing errors, we found—to our surprise—that the very best performer was the nuclear energy industry. Performance Improvement International (PII), a leading-edge company focused on improving human and organizational performance, turned out to have the very best methodology, and the best results. Beginning in the nuclear energy industry, PII has applied its breakthrough error reduction methodology in other energy industries and manufacturing with exceptional results. In fact, when PII applies its comprehensive assessment and implementation methodology in high-risk, complex organizations outside of health care, it has a demonstrated track record of achieving an 80% reduction in errors in just two years. Nothing comes close to this level of performance in health care.

The Greeley Company has been pleased to work with PII for the past several years in applying its exceptional methodology in health care. We are very excited with the progress we've made so far. Preliminary outcome results appear to suggest that health care can make the kinds of gains PII has helped nonhealth care organizations achieve.

An important part of PII's methodology includes conducting RCAs with exceptional discipline and skill, and using objective, reproducible tools health care has yet to discover. PII calls this approach "technology-based RCAs." The resulting RCAs are head-and-shoulders above anything we've seen in health care to date. Because of its exceptional reputation in performing RCAs, PII has been called upon to conduct more than 5,000 RCAs around the world in many different industries. Its results continue to be remarkably effective at identifying true root causes and what you will learn to call "root solutions." These are definitive, effective, and affordable corrective actions to prevent recurrences.

The Greeley Company and HCPro are very pleased to make PII's RCA methodology available to health care leaders through this extraordinary book, *Maximize Patient Safety with Advanced Root Cause Analysis*. Written by three partners at PII, these authors bring world-class knowledge and unparalleled experience in performing RCAs to this effort. I am sure this book will open your eyes to how much more the health care industry can gain from conducting a truly effective RCA. In fact, poorly performed RCAs cause health care organizations to spend time, energy, and resources working on the wrong things. The result is not only a waste of scarce resources, but ineffective changes that leave untouched the true root causes of errors that will continue to plague health care until we do something dramatically different.

## Applying RCA at your organization

As you will find in the pages of this book, health care leaders can readily carry out some of the methods of effective RCAs. Others will require more study and training, but it will be well worth the effort because of the valuable results they will produce. Some of the tools and methods described in this book may be beyond your organization's capabilities at this time. They are included both to challenge more advanced students of RCA and to help health care leaders catch a glimpse of the possibilities of what truly effective RCAs can accomplish.

Readers of this book are encouraged to adopt a "crawl-walk-run" approach to improving RCAs in their organizations. The first step—crawl—will help those responsible for conducting RCAs open their eyes to how much more effective our RCAs can be in improving safety and reducing errors if we learn and apply technology-based approaches. We hope you will carry out as many of the best practices for RCAs described in this book as possible during your crawl stage.

The second step is to make sure you adequately train those responsible for conducting RCAs in your organization to use many of the tools and approaches described in this book. This walk stage may require some time and resources. Your organization's leaders will inevitably ask about the return on investment (ROI) they can expect from significantly strengthening your RCAs. You can tell them that detection and correction technology-based RCA programs have been demonstrated to reduce losses from errors by 50% every two years in complex organizations in other high-risk industries. RCA does not contain all of the detection elements. Health care desperately needs approaches to reducing errors and improving patient safety that can deliver this kind of ROI.

Eventually, you may be able to lead your organization to the run stage. At that time you will leave most other health care organizations in the dust and dance circles around them with the quality and safety of the care you provide.

In the end, you conduct RCAs because someone in your organization has suffered an unnecessary injury or been exposed to the serious risk of such an injury. Conducting a good RCA that identifies true root solutions and prevents others from suffering the same injury is the very least we owe to the patients who entrust their care to us.

—*Richard* A. *Sheff*, MD, vice president of consulting and education at The Greeley Company, a division of HCPro.

# How to Use This Book

It is key for you to begin planning how to handle an event before it occurs. Start by taking the first step and then go one step at a time. Planning is the first step.

Take that first step now for two important reasons:

1. Because your organization needs the benefits received from a formal root cause analysis (RCA) program, including a 50% reduction in events within the first two years of implementation.[1]
2. Because the culture, infrastructure, skill sets, and processes needed to perform an effective RCA are not acquired overnight. Before you can expect to be successful in performing RCAs, you need to establish an effective infrastructure for the program.

If you are fortunate enough to work in an organization that has not recently experienced a sentinel event and you do not have an investigation that is urgent, take the time to learn what is needed to support RCAs and establish the infrastructure to support more effective RCA while you have the chance. By doing this, you will develop and implement a successful process—including working through potential pitfalls and challenges—before you experience a trigger event. In addition to reading this book, consider taking an RCA class or two. But most importantly, you should work with management to implement the policies, processes, forms, inservice packages, training classes, etc. needed to support this program.

## How management can support the process

Support from management is integral to successful implementation of RCAs. One of the most important actions management can take is to determine up-front what kinds of events will receive more formal investigation. This can eliminate the typical confusion about process and leadership that occurs when a decision is made in the heat of the moment, just after they receive notification of a serious event. It will also help improve the cost-effectiveness of carrying out RCAs. The result is greater ownership and support on the part of managers as they determine which events will warrant formal RCA

[1] Source: PII R&D Project: An Integrated Model for Event Rate Reduction from a Management Perspective, Performance Improvement International Technical Paper 95-542; Copyright, 1994.

investigations, and conversely, what kinds of issues are more efficiently resolved using less formal and unstructured problem-solving techniques. Once management decides what types of events will receive a particular level of investigation, this information must be captured to ensure a consistent response from the organization.

To address this need, other industries have used a problem initiation and screening matrix, which determines what types of issues warrant formal structured problem solving and the "level" of investigation to be applied for a particular type of event. This matrix was developed to trigger the organization to review external requirements and standards for the conduct of more thorough investigations (e.g., Joint Commission on Accreditation of Healthcare Organizations (JCAHO) standards for what constitutes a sentinel event) as well as state management expectations for the types of issues that should receive RCA.

As you prepare to implement more effective RCAs, remember that although the JCAHO has released some examples of what it means by "thorough and credible analysis of events," it has not specifically defined the criteria it will use to determine acceptable performance against this standard. Certainly, this will be an evolutionary process in health care, just as it has been for other high-risk industries that have gone down this road before.

## How this book is organized

This book provides a complete guide to the advanced RCA process:

- The introduction describes how you can reduce occurrences or events through prevention, detection, and correction of known causes and precursors.

- **Chapter 1** explains how RCA operates as a management function.

- **Chapter 2** provides an overview of the RCA process and the importance of conducting RCAs on nonsentinel events.

- **Chapter 3** instructs you on the first step of the process, investigating the event. It covers everything you need to know about your initial response to the event, beginning the investigation, and selecting the appropriate members for the RCA team.

- **Chapter 4** explains the second step—collecting data and information—and features how to turn raw information into facts.

- **Chapter 5** contains information on the third step—identifying the failure modes—such as equipment failures, inappropriate actions, and external events. It tells you how to identify possible causes and use appropriate diagnostic tools to aid in your investigation.

- **Chapter 6** walks readers through the fourth step, developing the failure scenarios. It explains attributes of a root cause, benchmarking, and how to handle multiple root causes of a single event.

- **Chapter 7** provides information about the fifth step, developing root solutions. It contains information about the differences between individual and system performance, why it's difficult to uncover a root solution, and how to effectively implement a corrective action.

- **Chapter 8** explains the final step in the process: monitoring for effectiveness. It explains the corrective action tracking system and the importance of using two tracking measures to obtain accurate monitoring results.

- **Chapter 9** describes the 25 elements of a high-performing cause-analysis program and how you can evaluate the effectiveness of your own program.

- **Chapter 10** explains how to go beyond RCAs to common-cause analyses. It also describes how and when to do an apparent-cause analysis for less significant events.

- The glossary (**Chapter 11**) contains essential terms used throughout the book. Make sure you review the glossary to fully understand the concepts discussed in each chapter.

- The appendices contain numerous tools, including a human error/inappropriate actions chart; organizational and programmatic diagnostic chart; and executive management failure mode chart.

This book can be your guide and key to successfully preparing for an RCA. After reading the chapters about how to conduct an investigation

- look over the sample charts and forms

- decide what you would use if you were responsible for conducting an important investigation starting tomorrow

- practice some of the basic RCA tools included in the Appendix

- review the forms—either use them as is or use them as a guide to create one for your own use

Preparation is the key to successful RCA; By reading this book, you are already on your way.

*Note:* We selected the following health care–specific example to demonstrate the need for formal root cause analysis (RCA).

**911 operator:** *"What is your emergency?"*
**Caller:** *"Please help us . . . she was unconscious, but now she screaming and crying . . . she keeps thrashing around in the bed . . . no one is helping us here . . . I think she's broken her arm too. Please, please help us!"*

**911 operator:** *"Who has broken their arm?"*

**Caller:** *"Our mother!"*

**911 operator:** *"What is your address?"*

**Caller:** *"Room 341, University Medical Center. We're in the new annex, please hurry."*

*Try to imagine the series of events that motivated this patient's family to seek help from 911-emergency assistance for their mother while she was in the care of a world-renowned hospital. Seems almost unimaginable doesn't it? How could a fairly routine and very successful operation result in such chaos?*

*What causes a family to panic to the point of calling for emergency medical technicians, when the experience and services of a giant research hospital are literally just down the hall? Let's explore the case study to see what prompted such extreme action.*

*The 62-year-old patient was the mother of five children. She had a long medical history that included six childbirths, a full hysterectomy at the age 26, osteo and rheumatoid arthritis, osteoporosis (brought on by the hysterectomy without hormone replacement), rheumatic fever that had weakened her heart muscle, congestive heart failure, and one heart attack. She had been operated on at this same facility, mostly under the care of the same physicians 24 times.*

*Due to the arthritis and osteoporosis, she has had both hips, both knees, and both elbows replaced. She underwent more than 30 surgical procedures by the time she had reached the age of 62. Her pain medicine regimen was extensive and dosages were systematically increased over the years to counteract the increasing pain throughout her arthritis-ravaged body. When old medications no longer provided at least tolerable relief to her pain, physicians ordered new, more potent medications. On average, she experienced two days per month in which she described her pain as tolerable.*

The patient was scheduled to have her left hip replaced for the second time. She received her first artificial hip 16 years earlier and it was now exhibiting wear-related problems. The surgeon who was scheduled to replace the hip had performed every one of her joint replacements. He was quite familiar with her medical history and had gained her trust and respect, as well as that of her family. Although the family was anxious about their mother undergoing yet another surgery, they felt reassured that who they considered the best surgeon and hospital staff available were conducting the procedure. Even their family physician was involved, as she always was when the woman was hospitalized. She even postponed her vacation until well after the surgery to personally follow her patient's progress. The surgery date was a consensus agreement among the patient, her family, the surgeon, and her primary care physician.

The patient was admitted to the hospital the evening before the surgery. The family and staff completed all necessary paperwork, including an exhaustive list of the 21 medications and dosages that made up the patient's daily regimen.

Some of the nursing staff had come to know the patient and her family personally, and came by to check on her even though they weren't assigned to her floor. The family requested a large room in the hospital's new VIP Annex, with windows overlooking a courtyard since they had stayed in that part of the building before.

At 12:15 p.m. the day after admission, the patient went into the operating room. By 4 p.m. the surgery was complete with no complications. The surgeon, smiling and vigorously shaking the hands of the family in the waiting room, was exuberant over the success of the surgery and the relative ease with which the patient seemed to tolerate the procedure.

The family breathed a collective sigh of relief and returned to the hospital room to await their mother's return from surgery. At this point, all appeared well and the family anticipated a smooth recovery.

At 5:30 p.m., 90 minutes after completion of the operation, the patient was wheeled into her private room in the annex and transferred to her bed. She initially appeared to be in almost no pain from the anesthetic. Although quite groggy, she was able to speak in short sentences. As the anesthetic began to wane, her pain level increased and she made this known to the family members in the room. At 5:45 p.m., the family summoned a nurse to the room to administer pain medication. The nurse responded and made a mental note that an infusion pump had not been set up. Upon returning to the nurse's station, she also noted that the pain medication indicated *by the pharmacy had not yet been drawn from supply. She began the process for acquiring the medication and equipment without returning to the family to explain this additional delay.*

*At 5:50 p.m., the patient was urgently vocalizing her pain with short muffled cries and labored breathing. By 6 p.m., the patient was in unbearable pain, screaming between gasps for air. Her daughter rushed to the nurse's station closest to her mother's room, but saw no one there. (The nurses were involved in shift turnover.) The patient's screams were heard at the station down the hall where one nurse was frantically working her way through the electronic process for drawing out the patient's prescribed medication.*

*At 6:30 p.m. the pain medication had still not been administered. The patient begged for a rag to bite down on. The family is near panic. Finally, after what seemed an eternity, a nurse arrives with an infusion pump and medication. After untangling the tubes and setting up the pump, a second nurse appeared and verified the infusion pump settings. At 6:45 p.m., the infusion pump was started and the family believed that pain relief was on the way.*

*However, by 7:10 p.m., the patient's pain had not moderated at all. Her son traced the intravenous (IV) lines and found a pinch clamp installed on the tube going into his mother's arm.*

*Her daughter rushed to the nurse's station again in a desperate attempt to locate the surgeon. She was informed that he was in surgery and wouldn't be available until after midnight, another five hours later. A nurse returned with the daughter to the patient's room to remove the pinch clamp. The family asked that nurses notify their family physician to come to the hospital immediately. They were concerned that all the stress of the operation and the out-of-control pain would be too much for their mother's heart. Her first heart attack resulted from very similar circumstances.*

*The patient screamed and thrashed her arms against the bed rails. Two nurses tried to apply restraints to control her movement, but not before she fractured her left arm.*

*Calls were made to the family physician, but her answering service referred all calls to the on-duty physician, who knew nothing about the patient's history and had not received turnover instructions regarding her case. As a result, he was unable to help.*

*Between the hours of 8 p.m. and 10 p.m., the patient alternated between periods of screaming and thrashing, and drifting in and out of consciousness. Providing too little relief, too late, the* minimal pain medication from the IV did not have any effect. When prompted to contact the pharmacy to increase her dosage, the nurses informed the family that only the surgeon could change the medication, and he would not available for another two hours.

After three more unsuccessful attempts to contact the family physician, and fearing for her mother's life due to the stress on her heart, the daughter dialed 911 from the third-floor hallway of the hospital and the operator dispatched emergency paramedics. As the paramedics began their emergency response, they quickly realized that they were responding to an emergency at the hospital that normally receives their patients.

Once the paramedics arrived at the patient's room, they told the family members there was nothing they could do. Hospital policy prevented them from providing medical care within the confines of the hospital.

Still reeling from the effects of their mother's condition and having to watch her suffer for more than six hours, family members momentarily consider moving her bed to the courtyard below.

At 12:30 a.m., the surgeon completed his surgical schedule and began final rounds to check on his patients. Upon arrival, he was informed of his patient's condition. Upon examination, he immediately doubled the dosage of her IV pain medication. He also added an order for additional injections, as needed, to control pain. By 2:15 a.m., the patient's pain began to moderate and she drifted into an uneasy sleep.

Based on information contained in the patient's chart, the surgeon ordered a lower right arm x-ray series to determine whether the arm was fractured. The following morning, the x-ray report indicated no fracture. When the family realized that the technicians x-rayed the wrong arm, they informed the surgeon. Much later that day, a technician x-rayed her left arm. This time, as expected, the x-ray indicated a fracture of the ulna.

Early the next morning, the local news media were covering the fiasco at the hospital after reviewing the previous night's 911 calls. They converged at the front door of the hospital lobby, clamoring for information related to the event. By 6 a.m., the hospital's main switchboard was jammed with incoming calls and the lobby was filled with cameras and field reporters all wanting to get the scoop. The hottest story of the year was a desperate 911-emergency call made by a patient's family member from the third floor of this very prestigious hospital.

**Note:** This isn't the first serious event to occur at a large, world-renowned research hospital, and it probably won't be the last. But the publicity created by this seemingly innocuous chain of events was the catalyst for the hospital to take actions that had far-reaching effects for the medical staff and the hospital leadership involved.

What caused this chain of events to spiral out of control? How did something that should have been a very routine function for this patient (administration of pain medication) go so terribly wrong? How could this happen, considering that previous surgeries at the same facility, with the same physicians, and the same medical staff, went so well?

As you'll discover in this book, single human errors rarely cause such significant events, even in complex, risk-averse organizations. But when multiple errors go undetected and uncorrected in a single system, and the cumulative impact of those errors weakens the organization's defenses— there is virtual certainty that they will trigger a chain of events so significant that even the strongest cannot prevail.

Does anyone think this event is just a simple case of human error and that there are not significant system issues that the organization needs to address? This book is designed to help you identify and correct the underlying causes of events like these.

# INTRODUCTION

## Improving Business Performance: Special Challenges in Complex Systems

# INTRODUCTION

---

# Improving Business Performance: Special Challenges in Complex Systems

## Adverse consequences—not human error—are the enemy

Adverse consequences and/or the potential for dangerous consequences define significant adverse events, such as sentinel events in hospitals. They are undesirable by definition and organizations continually strive to improve performance by reducing the frequency of significant events.

One hundred years ago, most events were caused by simple human errors. A single person could make a mistake that resulted in loss of life or property. As potential risks grew, society viewed them as too great and added more controls to systems so single human errors would be less likely to result in loss of life or property. These controls acted as barriers to prevent single human errors from resulting in significant events.

Today, single human errors rarely cause significant events. Modern systems have defense-in-depth in the form of multiple barriers to prevent events. So now when an organization experiences a significant event, there is virtual certainty that several causes acted together to both trigger the event and allow the failure of all of the barriers put in place to prevent the incident. For example, if a physician orders a medication that is contraindicated by other medications a patient is taking, there is a good chance that the pharmacist or the computerized order entry system will identify the concern before a nurse administers the medication. However, if these barriers also fail, the patient may suffer an adverse outcome.

---

## The Swiss cheese effect

Many people have described the idea of barriers as means to prevent events and barrier analysis as a method of cause analysis. However, no one has better described the initiation of the event and failure of barriers in the defense-in-depth of complex systems than Dr. James Reason in his later work, *Managing the Risks of Organizational Accidents.*[1]

Reason describes barriers as a series of defensive layers that allow no penetration by accident trajectories. When a barrier is weakened by an undesirable condition (i.e., degrading supervision or oversight), a "hole" develops in the barrier. If several holes develop in the defensive barriers, they begin to look like slices of Swiss cheese. These holes, which Reason called "latent conditions," can result in a pathway through the defenses that allows an inappropriate action or decision by individuals interfacing with the system to trigger a significant event.

Building on Reason's "Swiss cheese" model of defense, a concise approach to event investigation emerged. Since 1987, Performance Improvement International (PII) has used these concepts to investigate thousands of events in hundreds of organizations. We've organized the barriers in place to prevent unwanted events into the following three major areas:

- Individual human performance barriers
- Programmatic barriers
- Organizational/management barriers

Individual human performance barriers include adequate skills and knowledge, exercising good judgment, and paying attention to detail. Effective programmatic barriers include adequate level of procedural guidance, methods to report and resolve problems, appropriate levels of review, and verification of critical activities. Strong organizational and management barriers include a defined and controlled organization structure, appropriate allocation of resources, adequate management and team leader observations, effective risk identification and management, and the establishment of a strong organizational culture.

The figure on the next page illustrates the Reason model for significant events and the barrier analysis concepts as applied to a significant event. Therefore, internal factors (failures associated with a particular individual's performance) and external factors (resulting from organizational/programmatic deficiencies) generate significant events. The external factors constitute the majority of root causes of significant events (more than 85%).

---

[1] *Managing the Risks of Organizational Accidents,* Dr. James Reason, Ashgate Publishing Company, Brookfield, VT, 1997.

---

| Figure I.1 | | **The Swiss cheese effect** | |

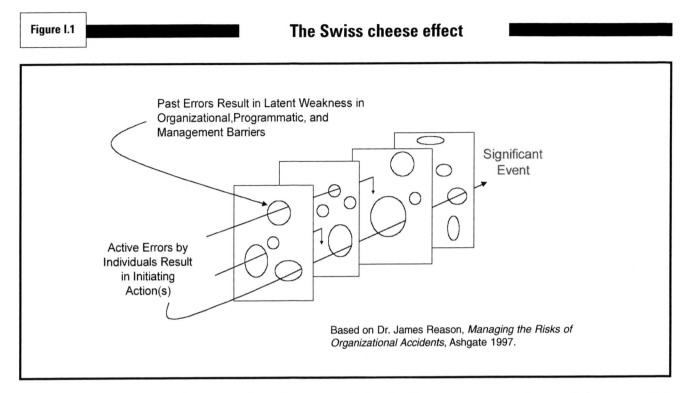

Past Errors Result in Latent Weakness in Organizational, Programmatic, and Management Barriers

Significant Event

Active Errors by Individuals Result in Initiating Action(s)

Based on Dr. James Reason, *Managing the Risks of Organizational Accidents*, Ashgate 1997.

The Swiss cheese model is an excellent illustration of why significant events occur in complex systems. But what causes the human error that initiates the event? Drs. Richard Cook and David Wood explain it in a model they refer to as "The Sharp End,"[2] which describes a complex system that provides a large set of behavior-shaping factors that are often competing.

The complex system is the blunt end. The health care provider at the sharp end continuously makes comprises when real-life situations conflict with the ideal action defined by the system. Most of the compromises are successful and ensure patient safety. Occasionally, a compromise is not successful and it creates an error and diminishes patient safety. The behavior-shaping factors in the blunt end are often found to be "causes" of the error in the system.

## Five-point philosophy

This background discussion leads us to an important question: If significant adverse events result from individual human errors and organizational/programmatic breakdowns, what philosophy must we use to reduce the likelihood of these events? Many previous clients began their performance improvement initiatives by adopting the following, basic five-point philosophy for human performance improvement and human error reduction:

[2]Cook R, Woods D (1994) *Operating at the Sharp End: The Complexity of Human Error.* In Bognar, MS, ed. Human Error in Medicine. Hillsdale, NJ: Lawrence Erlbaum, pp. 255-310.

**1.** All people—even highly skilled, knowledgeable, and successful professionals—make errors. Therefore, in a higher risk environment, an organization does not allow, nor depend on, the individual performer to be the only barrier against events.

**2.** Error-likely, or high-risk situations are predictable, manageable, and preventable. (See the Appendix for "The top 12 high-risk situations causing sentinel events in health care.")

**3.** Individual behavior is strongly influenced by organizational, programmatic, and management performance or the organization's "culture." In other words, an organization's "culture" in an organization strongly influences the behaviors of the individuals in that organization. Their behaviors thus determine performance outcomes—good or bad.

**4.** High-risk behaviors result in human errors or inappropriate actions that trigger events. (See the Appendix for "The top 12 high-risk behaviors causing sentinel events in health care.") Conversely, an organization can achieve optimum levels of human performance (few human errors) if they encourage, teach, and reinforce appropriate behavior.

**5.** Organizations can avoid significant events by understanding and monitoring precursor conditions (i.e., near misses) and by applying lessons learned from past significant events through rigorous root cause analysis (RCA).

## Sentinel events in health care

Medical errors and sentinel events are not new in hospitals. In fact, they have been occurring for as long as hospitals have existed. These mistakes were generally accepted as an inevitable consequence of the complex and high-risk activities inherent in caring for sick patients. However, with the introduction of continuous performance-improvement approaches in health care, the industry began to see the analysis of sentinel and other adverse events as a tool for improving processes and outcomes. Such an approach requires that when a sentinel event occurs, an organization performs an analysis to identify proximate causes of the event and then takes actions to prevent these from recurring.

However, organizations soon discovered that addressing only the proximate causes leads to a likelihood that a similar event could occur elsewhere. Therefore, to achieve the maximum value from the analysis of an adverse event, high-performing organizations now go beyond proximate causes to identify true root causes and generic implications. By identifying and addressing root causes, an organization is best able to prevent a recurrence of similar events throughout the facility.

Other industries, such as nuclear energy and aviation embraced this approach several years ago. In fact, these industries also found that performing common-cause analyses on many "near misses" and then an RCA on the identified common causes, led to improvements that prevented future tragedies.

## Error reduction through Prevention, Detection, Correction

Given this background, how can an organization systematically improve the human performance of its staff? PII's research and case studies indicate the most effective event and human error reduction programs focus on prevention of errors, detection of event precursors, and correction of event causes. This Prevention, Detection, and Correction (PDC™) strategy is described in more detail below.

**Prevention** (P) of events and human errors takes place by

- establishing mission, goals, and behavior-based expectations consistent with high management standards for event-free performance

- educating individuals at all levels in the organization on comprehensive error prevention techniques

- establishing an effective accountability system to ensure people comply with behavior-based expectations and use the error-prevention techniques.

**Detection** (D) of precursors before they cause significant events by

- conducting periodic organizational, programmatic, and management error common-cause analyses, or performance monitoring, to determine underlying precursors to human error

- making effective use of "leading," "real-time," and "lagging" performance indicators, or performance trending, to determine if current and future performance is and will be acceptable

- implementing effective internal (i.e., quality assurance) and external oversight

- using in-house and industry lessons learned and self-assessments.

**Correction** (C) of events (e.g., to prevent recurrence) by

- using strong human-error, organizational, and programmatic diagnostic and corrective action capabilities of line managers and root cause investigators

- creating an effective, integrated problem-reporting, resolution, and action tracking system.

An integrated approach to performance improvement is critical. When D and C are poor, the event rate will actually increase as poorly crafted corrective actions make the processes and organizations more error-prone. When D and C are good, the event rate decreases, although the time frame to realize the performance improvement is long because both detection and correction are "event-based". Prevention of errors is the most cost-effective method of performance improvement. However, without effective D and C the organization will be overly dependent on people as the last line of defense. Therefore, integrated P, D, and C are necessary for rapid and sustained event rate reduction.

The PDC approach requires involvement at all levels in the organization. Specific initiatives must be in place to prevent events, detect event precursors, and correct the causes of events. This integrated approach is illustrated in Figure I.2 on the next page. While a major focus of this book is on improving patient safety and reducing the number of sentinel events through effective RCA, organizations need to realize that these efforts also result in improved quality, cost, satisfaction, and productivity. The PDC-approach is more than a safety improvement program. It's an integrated performance improvement program that reduces the likelihood of human errors and process breakdowns.

RCA is a key initiative under the "correction" column in the figure on the next page and is the primary topic of this book. The reader should be aware that many other activities beyond RCA are included in a comprehensive and integrated performance improvement initiative.

Before we begin to discuss advanced methods of cause analysis, it's important to understand key terms and discuss several important concepts. You'll find a complete list of these definitions in Chapter 11.

| Figure I.2 | An Integrated Approach to Prevention, Detection, Correction (PDC) |

| | Prevention Initiatives | Detection Initiatives | Correction Initiatives |
|---|---|---|---|
| Management Systems | ✓ | ✓ | ✓ |
| Organizational & Programmatic Systems | ✓ | ✓ | ✓ |
| Individual Work Practices | ✓ | ✓ | ✓ |

# CHAPTER 1

## Root Cause Analysis is a Management Function

# CHAPTER 1

---

# Root Cause Analysis is a Management Function

The next time you walk into a bookstore, make it a point to visit the business section. It seems that on a near hourly basis, a new book describes some trendy, need-to-have-it management theory or concept that will produce remarkable results when incorporated in your daily approach to business. Texts describing management functions could fill a small library. Yet, in all studies and analyses of management performance, one major theme consistently appears: management's job is to control performance to achieve desired outcomes.

Simply put, the purpose of management is to perform the following four functions:

1. **Plan** the conduct of activities

2. **Organize** resources and processes to execute the plan

3. **Direct** the implementation of the activity

4. **Control** the entire process by monitoring output, comparing results to expectations, and making necessary adjustments

It is the fourth bullet (control) that most closely ties the root cause analysis (RCA) process to management's function.

Figure 1.1 illustrates these four functions.

---

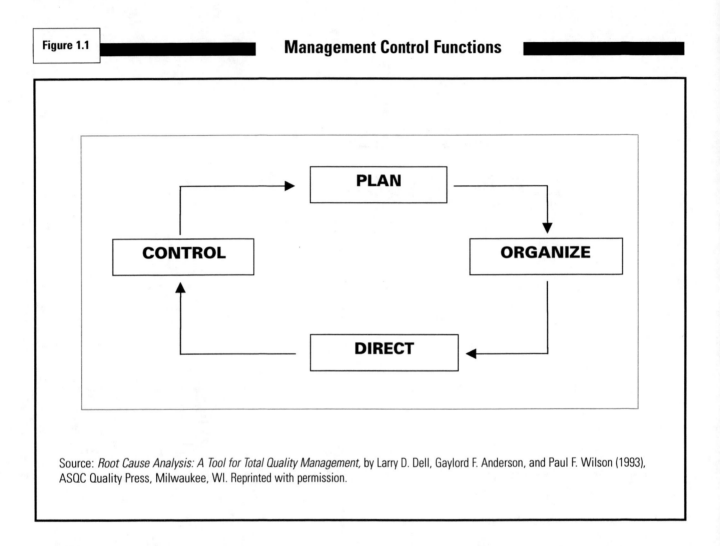

**Figure 1.1** ████████ **Management Control Functions** ████████

PLAN

CONTROL

ORGANIZE

DIRECT

Source: *Root Cause Analysis: A Tool for Total Quality Management,* by Larry D. Dell, Gaylord F. Anderson, and Paul F. Wilson (1993), ASQC Quality Press, Milwaukee, WI. Reprinted with permission.

## Controlling phase

The controlling phase involves determining the effectiveness of performance by measuring and comparing results against expectations. If results meet these expectations, management does not need to make corrective adjustments. But if results don't meet expectations, managers must make adjustments. Smart managers will perform a cause analysis to determine the reason for the gap (see Figure 1.2 on the next page).

In cases where the gap represents a serious deficiency, managers should perform an RCA to determine the cause of the problem. The RCA process will reveal the cause of shortcomings embedded in standards, expectations, procedures, processes, and personnel behaviors. These shortcomings represent weaknesses, referred to in the introduction as "latent conditions or holes in the Swiss cheese" that management must fix. As shown in Figure 1.2, the management control loop provides feedback to the organization about how well corrective actions have worked to improve the performance and prevent repeat failure.

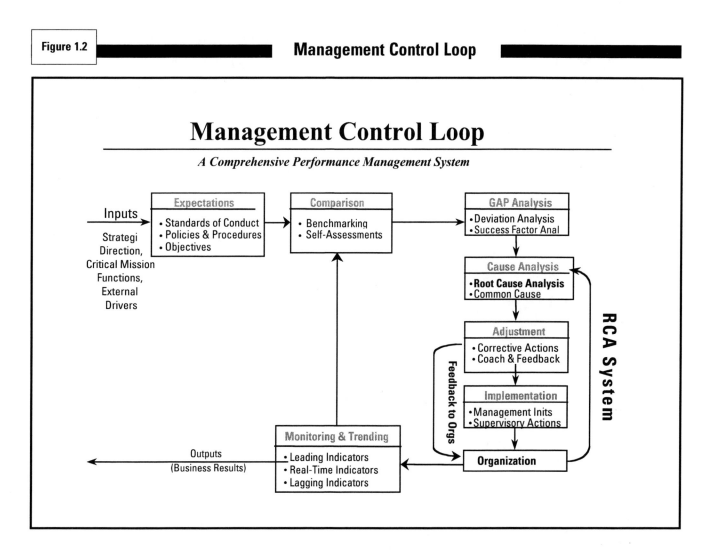

**Figure 1.2**     Management Control Loop

In order for these adjustments to work, managers must take responsibility for the RCA process and own the resulting recommendations for improvement. This means managers must accept and support the recommendations offered by root cause investigators. An apathetic or aggressive response could stop the process entirely. Employees selected to investigate events in this culture quickly learn what topics are off limits and will work hard to avoid traveling into management quicksand.

## RCA is a management function, performed by staff

Although line management sponsors and leads the RCA process, the organization assigns staff to conduct investigations. Whoever is assigned to the team must be careful not to use RCA as a weapon for justifying disciplinary action and other punitive responses toward employees who are involved in events.

In truth, PII's research, as well as that of other experts[3], has repeatedly shown that although individual human error may have triggered an event, organizational and management weaknesses allowed the individual error to escalate into more serious consequences and events 85% of the time. (Refer to the introduction and the discussion regarding the Swiss cheese model from Dr. James Reason.)

In order to be effective, an organization must accept that the result of any given RCA is for improvement—rather than assignment of blame. This is in keeping with the basic philosophy and tenet of continuous improvement in any area of endeavor.

One area of undisputed agreement is that without strong support from upper management, health care organizations will perform RCA in a perfunctory manner with the singular purpose of meeting the Joint Commission on Accreditation of Healthcare Organization's (JCAHO) standards.

Another challenge facing health care management is that it must actively motivate those who serve on the team. Employees must experience the rewards of following the process early and have leaders view their participation in a positive light. Otherwise, the process is destined to fail.

## Summary

A healthy root cause program exists when staff and employees readily participate by reporting minor errors, precursor incidents, improvement needs, and events. Then RCA teams can analyze reported items and solve problems using RCA to produce effective corrective actions. The organization can carry out corrective actions and monitor the process to make sure the desired change occurs.

With this process effectively in place and thriving in a professional environment, the performance of the individuals and the organization as a whole will steadily and measurably improve. Personnel will spend less time agonizing over and reacting to failures, and more time improving their performance and ultimately, the standard of care provided to patients. It is the very best kind of win-win.

---

[3]Dr. Edwards Deming reported that up to 90% of all events are caused by management and system failures.

---

# CHAPTER 2

# Overview of the Root Cause Analysis Process

# Overview of the Root Cause Analysis Process

The root cause of an event is defined as the most basic condition in a failure scenario that, if eliminated, would prevent recurrence of an event. A thorough and credible root cause analysis (RCA) is the result of a process that provides the framework and structure to

- evaluate adverse events or conditions
- determine root cause(s)
- develop comprehensive corrective actions to preclude recurrence

The six steps outlined in this chapter provide a repeatable, defendable process that meets and surpasses the challenge from the Joint Commission on Accreditation of Healthcare Organizations (JCAHO) to be thorough and credible. Other high-risk/high-complexity organizations have successfully used this process to significantly reduce undesirable incidents by as much as 50% in a two-year period. Further, no matter what the industry or the event that drives the need for RCA, the basic process does not change.

## Roadmap for the RCA process

*Note to readers: Use the figure on the next page to guide your review of the six steps in Performance Improvement International's (PII's) Advanced RCA process. This chapter provides an introduction and an overview of the six steps. Chapters 3–8 offer detailed guidance on each step in the process. This roadmap provides a quick reference to the location of detailed guidance within the book and a reminder as to where in the book each step falls.*

Figure 2.1    **Roadmap of the Root Cause Analysis Process**

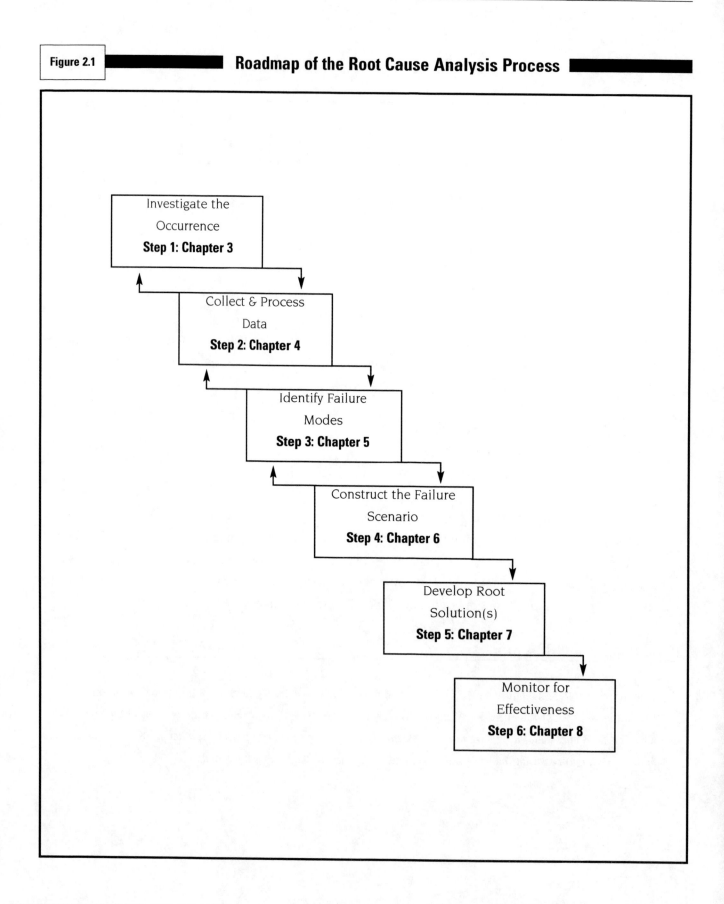

Investigate the
Occurrence
**Step 1: Chapter 3**

Collect & Process
Data
**Step 2: Chapter 4**

Identify Failure
Modes
**Step 3: Chapter 5**

Construct the Failure
Scenario
**Step 4: Chapter 6**

Develop Root
Solution(s)
**Step 5: Chapter 7**

Monitor for
Effectiveness
**Step 6: Chapter 8**

An RCA should be a consistent process anchored in sound technology. Organizations can easily trace the steps performed in an RCA because the report includes the results of each step. An organization can easily repeat the process over time to produce consistent, high-quality results from investigations of important events.

Root cause analysts function for their organizations as doctors do for their patients: they diagnose their organizations' "illnesses" and prescribe corrective measures to cure the problem with minimal negative "side effects."

## Six steps to the finish line

The RCA process developed by PII provides organizations with a structured approach that uses commonly found RCA "tools" to complete investigations in a logical, methodical order. As a result of 40,000 case studies and more than 5,000 RCA investigations performed by PII to date, PII has boiled down the entire RCA process into the six simple steps provided in this text. (See Figure 2.2.)

The following section provides an overview of the six steps. **Chapters 3-8** present more detailed guidance on the individual RCA steps.

So, where do you start?

### Step 1: Investigate the occurrence
Every RCA begins with an investigation, beginning as soon as possible after an organization learns of the event. The old saying "time changes everything" is certainly true, especially when it relates to the memory of individuals involved in an event. It is a typical human response to confuse actual conditions and actions that *did* occur with what the mind believes *should have* occurred. See **Chapter 3** for more information on how to investigate the event.

### Step 2: Collect and process information
The next logical step in the RCA process involves gathering data and evidence to support a review of the inappropriate actions identified and how they might have occurred. Physical evidence, documentation, personal statements, instrumentation output (strip charts and recorder data), and programmatic guidance are all common sources of information. Again, time is of the essence. Collecting data and information as close to the actual occurrence of the event as possible will minimize the potential for the normal atrophy of memory that comes with the passage of time. See **Chapter 4** for details on how to collect and process information.

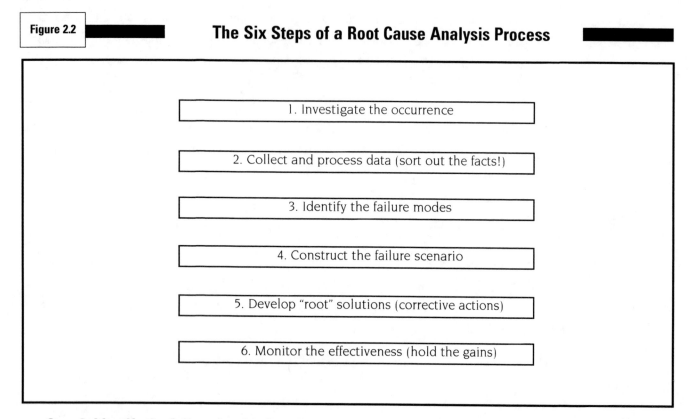

**Figure 2.2          The Six Steps of a Root Cause Analysis Process**

1. Investigate the occurrence

2. Collect and process data (sort out the facts!)

3. Identify the failure modes

4. Construct the failure scenario

5. Develop "root" solutions (corrective actions)

6. Monitor the effectiveness (hold the gains)

### Step 3: Identify the failure mechanisms

The goal of this step of the process is to identify the most basic condition(s) that caused the event (failure mechanisms). Once we determine the facts surrounding the incident, we can begin to identify potential failure mechanisms and note them as such in the evidence matrix. PII recommends using a *technology-based* approach when performing RCA to ensure that your organization considers all known failure modes. *"Technology-based"* refers to the use of specific root cause diagnostic charts and information. Organizations use the diagnostic charts to identify all possible failure modes for a particular incident or inappropriate action. The correlation between observed symptoms and specific failure modes is supported through our rigorous research of case studies and adverse event data. See **Chapter 5** for more information on this step in the process.

### Step 4: Construct the failure scenario (piece together the story)

Once we identify the probable failure mechanisms through facts, evidence, and information collected to support our hypotheses; we are ready to construct the failure scenario. This part of the RCA process involves constructing the "story" that explains what happened in the event. The failure scenario summarizes the cause(s), the sequence of events, and their connection to the consequences of incident.

The failure scenario (Figure 2.2) briefly describes the event, connecting the cause to the consequences, in both a visual and a narrative format.

This makes it easier for those not involved in the event to understand what occurred. See **Chapter 6** for more information on constructing the failure scenario.

### Step 5: Identify and carry out "root solutions."

Just as the goal of Step 3 of the RCA process is to identify the most basic condition(s) that caused the event, the focus of this step of the process is to determine the most basic corrective action(s) that will prevent recurrence of the event. We refer to these actions as "root solutions."

The following are the three types of corrective actions resulting from an RCA:

1. **Remedial actions** ("broke-fix" actions, taken right away to correct the immediate damage)
2. **Interim compensatory actions** (measures taken to limit the possibility of further damage or recurrence in the short term)
3. **Preventive actions**, also known as corrective actions to prevent recurrence or CATPR (taken to ensure long-term prevention of recurrence)

---

### A health care example

*A 55-year-old man presents to the emergency department with escalating episodes of substernal chest pain without EKG or enzyme changes. The physician diagnoses unstable angina. The physician takes **remedial actions** that include prescribing oxygen and nitroglycerine. The patient's pain subsides and he is transferred to the hospital's coronary care unit. As part of the diagnostic work-up, the cardiologist performs a cardiac catheterization, identifying one severe coronary artery blockage and several less-severe blockages. The cardiologist provides interim relief (**interim compensatory actions**) by performing angioplasty and stent placement for the severe blockage. This treatment will temporarily limit recurrence of the angina. However, given this patient's age and the other developing blockages, life-threatening angina is likely to recur unless the cardiologist takes **preventive actions** to eliminate the root causes of his predisposition for atherosclerosis. Appropriate corrective actions to prevent recurrence (CATPR) must address the root cause of his angina. These will include prescription of lipid lowering agents, dietary changes, and regular exercise.*

This example is particularly appropriate because it demonstrates the importance of following through and identifying corrective actions to prevent recurrence, both in the practice of medicine for the patient and the conduct of RCA for the organization. In both instances, preventive actions will only be effective if the "patient" consistently follows through. Failure to follow through with implementing CATPR—identified during an RCA is a common problem in hospitals. See **Chapter 7** for more information on identifying root solutions.

---

### Step 6: Monitor for effectiveness

The last step in the RCA process establishes a control loop to make sure that the results of the analysis produce the desired outcome. This involves tracking the corrective actions through to completion, ensuring that performance improves as intended, and monitoring in the future to ensure repeat or similar events do not recur. See **Chapter 8** for more information on how to monitor for effectiveness.

## Knowledge and skill sets for root cause analysts

Every organization is composed of employees with varying degrees of education, skill, and experience. Your goal is to find the members who have a combination of necessary qualities to serve on the RCA team.

Some members are known for their natural troubleshooting and problem-solving abilities (the first skill set needed to support effective RCA). No matter their background or experience, they seem to have the intuition and natural ability to ask the right questions and navigate layers of complexity to identify the one or two issues most likely to have caused the event in question. These are the individuals who the organization turns to when a crisis occurs. They ride in on white horses, troubleshoot the problem, and like the heroes in good western movies, restore calm and ride off into the sunset.

Others in the organization are subject-matter experts or "specialists" (the second type of knowledge needed to support effective problem solving). These individuals specialize in one particular subject or area, spending years studying the depths of their chosen field, and over time learn all there is to know about the topic. They also support their organizations by providing expert opinions for correcting maladies within their respective disciplines.

It takes both skill sets to achieve the desired outcome in performing RCA. After all, what good are phenomenal troubleshooters if they don't know all the possible failures to troubleshoot? And conversely, how much help can subject matter experts provide if they understand all of the intricate nuances of a particular system, but they can't put that knowledge to use in a systematic diagnosis of the problem?

Expert root cause analysts may possess an equal share of each strength. It is more likely that the organization will find the knowledge and skills needed to effectively perform an RCA in the combination and collective makeup of the team of individuals assigned to solve a specific performance problem.

Medical professionals must also possess both types of expertise. They spend years in higher education to obtain the textbook knowledge of how the human body works and how failure manifests itself. They follow up their formal education with years of practice, applying diagnostic skills in combination with the knowledge of possible failures (causes for illness or malady) to effectively treat patients.

The very best RCA teams include a combination of good "organization doctors," who possess effective problem-solving and failure-diagnosing skills; and credible, capable, and medical subject matter experts, selected for their knowledge of areas applicable to the event of interest. The combination of these critical components (expert problem solvers and credible subject matter experts) is a powerful weapon in a health care organization's battle to remain fiscally sound and operationally competitive.

## Justification for performing a formal RCA

In cases where symptoms point to a definitive ailment, a medical professional may make a quick judgment as to the cause of the problem (diagnosis) and choose to treat the condition with a similarly routine regimen. In most cases, good results ensue and the patient is on the road to recovery. However, some symptoms, due to their frequency, severity, recurrence rate, etc., may indicate another underlying problem that requires treatment. Until that underlying condition is known and corrected, the symptoms will likely recur, increasing in frequency and intensity.

This analogy underscores the need to look beyond the first diagnosis of symptoms evidenced in an event and conduct a more thorough review (investigation) into the cause of the symptoms. The following example reinforces this point:

*A female patient is diagnosed by her family physician with a urinary tract infection (UTI). A course of antibiotics clears her symptoms. However, over the next two years, this patient receives five additional treatments for UTIs: two by her family physician, one by a physician at a vacation resort hotel, and two treatments at an urgent care clinic. When the patient returns to her family physician for a sixth treatment, the doctor asks her about the complete history of the infection. After learning that other health care providers rendered additional treatments, and based on the increased frequency and severity of the infections, her physician determines that he needs to conduct additional tests. A cystoscopy reveals a mass on the bladder wall. When surgically removed, the mass proves to be a foreign body left behind when the patient underwent bladder repair surgery six years earlier. After the foreign body is removed, the patient's health improves and the occurrence of UTIs returns to a normal frequency.*

This case study represents what can happen when a caregiver treats symptom(s) of a problem, but the underlying cause of the symptom(s) remains undetected. The same analogy holds true for investigating the cause of organizational events. To ensure you effectively address significant or recurring problems in the performance of individuals, processes, and systems within the organization, you must systematically evaluate observed problems and conditions, determine their root causes, carry out corrective actions, and then monitor the effectiveness of the actions taken.

The more common approaches for identifying root causes in health care have relied heavily on profession-al experience and seasoned judgment to find the "smoking gun" when an incident occurred. In many cases, years of education, practical knowledge, and the experience of individuals merged successfully to lead to effective diagnosis of a performance problem, and organizations took effective actions to prevent recurrence. For just this reason, we all take great comfort knowing that medical professionals are excep-tionally well educated and routinely share knowledge and experience through consultation to diagnose and treat patients. But not all patients are this fortunate or are all caregivers equal in professional knowl-edge or ability.

In fact, the unstructured methods used in lieu of RCA are partially to blame for number of events that are repeated in the health care industry. It is for this very reason that the JCAHO has instituted guidelines to improve the conduct of RCA investigations across the industry. In our own review of significant event analyses conducted by health care organizations, we found these reviews to be subjective, limited in their review of potential causes (not comprehensive), and at times intentionally vague. This is true especially when all of the pertinent information is not known or unavailable to individuals involved in the analysis. It is also the case when analysts involved in the review do not represent all fields of knowledge and expert-ise needed to investigate and solve the problem.

A more structured RCA process ensures that organizations accurately identify and conclusively analyze adverse conditions. By doing so, organizations can then identify corrective actions that will solve serious problems with a high degree of reliability, and prevent future recurrence.

## Implementing the six-step process through the 'Three-Meeting Model'

When conducting an RCA, it is essential that you use an efficient, effective structure to facilitate comple-tion of the six steps in the investigation process: efficient, so that time-sensitive information is not lost and the cost of conducting the investigation is acceptable to the organization; effective, so that the inves-tigation results in root solutions that prevent recurrence. One technique used in the health care industry to meet this challenge is called the "Three-Meeting Model."

The Three-Meeting Model is as simple as the name implies. Using PII's six-step RCA process, organiza-tions can complete the activities included in each of the steps within three (or four, if needed) meetings of the RCA team. Each meeting takes two to three hours to complete. By the conclusion of these meetings, the team should have reached consensus on the cause of the event and developed corrective action recommendations for improvement.

Using this approach, an organization appoints a qualified RCA facilitator to coordinate the investigation process and complete actions in preparation for each meeting. The role of this individual is critical since the outcome will depend largely on the effectiveness of planning and preparation for each meeting and the quality of information the facilitator provides to the team. (In some organizations, this person is referred to as the team leader. In others, team leader and facilitator are separate positions on the RCA team.) When selecting the facilitator, senior leaders in the organization should choose someone experienced in the conduct of RCAs. This person may or may not be familiar with the event requiring investigation.

In many health care facilities, the risk manager or quality manager (or a similar staff position) is appointed to function in this role for all RCA investigations. Although there is no doubt that it is convenient for senior leadership to know they have a designated position (and therefore individual) to perform this function, it can also be limiting.

By always looking to the same individual to serve as the RCA team leader, organization leaders limit the number of employees who gain experience and proficiency in overseeing this function. In many of the cases we have reviewed, the risk manager became the individual who performed most of the investigative work while the "team" simply rubber-stamped the results. This serves as a second limiting factor by minimizing the number of employees who actually become qualified in the RCA process.

A better arrangement is to have the risk manager act as a true facilitator of the process. In this role, the facilitator directs another individual, selected to act as the team leader, through the process. The team leader may be a manager or another key player in the group affected by the incident, or may be a star player who needs additional challenges and career development. In either case, by naming a separate party to act as a team leader, the organization improves the bench strength of individuals qualified to lead RCA investigations. (A nice side effect of doing this is the increase in buy-in and ownership for RCA felt by individuals in key positions within the organization.)

Team members should represent a cross-section of disciplines and groups. Usually no more than two to four people are needed as team members. Team members should include some individuals who are knowledgeable about the incident and some who are not knowledgeable (and are therefore unbiased).

The facilitator (or team leader being mentored) conducts the three meetings, incorporating the associated root cause steps as noted on the next page. (These steps are further described in **Chapters 3–8.**) Prior to and between meetings, the facilitator (or team leader) should make sure that the group receives and completes action assignments to support upcoming meeting objectives and key decision points.

### RCA Meeting #1

Purpose: To familiarize the team with the event, analyze the problem, and recommend immediate compensatory actions to management, if required.

*Steps 1, 2, and 3 of the PII RCA process support the objectives of the first meeting. At this meeting the entire team analyzes the information collected and works as a group to identify potential failure mechanisms for further review. Remedial and compensatory actions are recommended, based on observed symptoms.*

### RCA Meeting #2

Purpose: To determine the cause of the problem and identify any significant contributing factors.

*The balance of Step 3 and all of Step 4 of the PII RCA process supports the objective of the second meeting in this model. At this meeting the team revises its failure scenario as needed based on previous actions to validate and verify its information. The team then identifies and reaches consensus as to the root cause(s) and key contributing factors of the event.*

### RCA Meeting #3

Purpose: To finalize the draft report (including recommendations for actions to prevent recurrence) and develop a plan to review effectiveness in the future.

*Steps 5 and 6 of the PII RCA process support the objectives of the final meeting. During this meeting, the team reaches consensus on information contained in the final (draft) report to management, including the following:*

- *Stated root cause(s) and key contributing factors*
- *Actions to prevent recurrence of root cause(s) and key contributing factors*
- *Actions to address generic implications*
- *A plan to review effectiveness of actions in the future*

The facilitator should schedule all team meetings in advance to allow all participants to attend.

## Conducting RCA on nonsentinel events

The health care industry began performing RCAs because of the JCAHO requirement to perform thorough and credible investigations for all sentinel events. This led to an assumption that teams must conduct RCAs for all events and the process would consume significant resources and time. This is true for investigations of catastrophic events that kill or severely injure patients and those that meet the definition of 'sentinel event'. Individual root cause investigators should also apply the six-step RCA process outlined in this book as they analyze the cause of events that are serious, but do not rise to the level of a sentinel event.

Using the RCA techniques presented in this book to identify and correct the root causes of less significant, but serious events will not only improve performance in those areas, but will contribute to your ability to prevent the occurrence of future sentinel events. In fact, outside the health care industry, organizations with strong safety and prevention cultures perform RCAs on events that fall just below the threshold for the equivalent of a sentinel-type event.

## Summary

The motivation to conduct more structured RCAs in health care is easily found in the imperative to reduce errors and the desire to remain fiscally competitive. In addition, a medical misadventure with a poor outcome could easily invite a malpractice suit from an injured patient or an angry survivor.

A credible and thorough RCA can be very valuable in planning for the defense of a malpractice suit against a practitioner/health care organization. In addition, an effective RCA can help mitigate the losses associated with professional liability claims.

High-quality RCAs also add value for the legal teams charged with preparing and presenting a defense for the accused hospital or medical provider. (Believe it or not, we have even observed hospital attorneys encouraging the performance of an RCA in response to an adverse event or outcome.)

Ultimately, the structured approach to RCA represented in the six steps outlined in this book, can minimize the pain felt by those assigned to perform investigations in your organization and effectively eliminate the guesswork that characterized the less formal and unstructured problem-solving methods used in the past.

The process we use here is based on facts, supported by a healthy level of rigor, and anchored in sound technology. It provides a direct path to success, ultimately delivering "root solutions" and the peace of mind that comes from knowing that we can prevent recurrence of failures in the future. After all, continuing to experience preventable failure is NOT an option when the basis of the oath and commitment made is to "First do no harm."

# CHAPTER 3

## Investigate
## the Event

# CHAPTER 3

# Investigate the Event

## STEP 1

## Introduction

If you are an investigator assigned to an organization that has experienced a sentinel event or a series of events, and you have to perform formal root cause analyses (RCAs) now with no time to prepare, you are likely functioning in crisis mode as you struggle to recover. Your challenge is difficult, but not unachievable.

Hopefully you have planned for how you'll handle an adverse event. (See "How to Use This Book" for more information.) This chapter details your next step: how to investigate an event. Subsequent chapters walk you through each step that follows the investigation.

In this chapter, you'll learn the first three parts of the investigative process:

1. First response
2. Gathering the RCA team
3. Beginning the investigation

## First response to an event

Your hospital has experienced an event. An RCA team is called into action, as are you. Right away you're asking the following questions:

- Who makes the first call?
- How does the investigation actually start?
- Who authorizes the allocation of resources and personnel?

Before you can even respond to these questions, follow the instructions listed below

### Seven steps to follow immediately after notification of an event

1) Take immediate action to protect people (patients and employees), equipment, and the environment. Use quarantine procedures where needed to prevent contamination of evidence and minimize disruption at the site.

2) Protect and preserve evidence.

3) Notify management and outside agencies (as required).

4) Use your organization's problem-reporting system to submit the incident for screening and potential analysis.

5) Identify the people who were involved in or observed the event and get a statement from them as soon as possible once safe conditions are restored. (The Appendix provides a sample form for this purpose.)

6) Select a management sponsor and an RCA team leader. They should immediately begin developing the problem statement.

7) Define the incident. A problem may be evidenced by
   - a deviation from normal practice, requirement, or expectations
   - an undesirable event, situation, or performance trend

### Prior to the first RCA team meeting, create a problem statement

A careful, clear, and specific problem statement saves time and focuses your investigative efforts. (See the Appendix for a sample form.) After you complete your problem statement, perform a check to see whether your problem is well defined. You should be able to answer, "yes" to all the following questions:

❑ Does my problem statement focus on the gap between "what is" and "what should be"?

❑ Does my problem statement communicate the effect, not the presumed cause?

❑ Does my problem statement communicate what appears to be wrong?

❑ Does my problem statement define (if applicable) how often, how much, and when?

❑ Is my problem statement communicated in a positive manner?

❏ Does my problem statement avoid "lack of" and "no" statements?

❏ Does my problem statement contain "no" solutions or conclusions?

❏ Is my problem statement as specific as possible?

Correct any problems or deficiencies in your problem statement.

## Gather the RCA team—a guide to who should be included

When selecting RCA team members, diversity is the key. The more varied the backgrounds and experience, the better the team seems to work together.

RCA team members should come from a cross-section of groups represented by the event of interest. They may or may not have been previously exposed to RCA. There should be at least one individual on the team who is a subject matter expert for the event of interest.

As soon as possible after being named, the responsible management sponsor should meet with the RCA team to discuss and agree upon the scope and objectives of the RCA. Sometimes this has to be a repetitive process based on the initial investigation results. Resources allocated to the investigation should be adjusted accordingly.

Not all evaluations will require or need a team effort. The need for a team v. a single individual should be assessed and determined by the responsible sponsor. In general, it is better to have two or more individuals working on an issue. For some issues, it is desirable to include expertise from the various departments involved. (Specific knowledge and skills for RCA team members are discussed in **Chapter 1**, "RCA is a management function, performed by staff.")

The following paragraphs discuss the different positions on the RCA team.

### *Management sponsor*
The management sponsor is selected by senior leadership to act as a liaison between management and the RCA team for the duration of the investigation. This individual is responsible for making sure the RCA team has adequate resources, support, cooperation, and time to perform their investigation.

One of the management sponsor's first responsibilities is to provide a management-approved problem statement for the investigation to the RCA team leader.

### *Team leader and RCA process facilitator*

The management sponsor will likely appoint an RCA team leader and a process facilitator. The team leader is not always RCA-qualified, but rather is a subject matter expert on the topic of the investigation or within the group that is the subject of the review.

The facilitator is the RCA process expert who will guide the team (and the team leader) through the investigation.

The team leader and the facilitator should sit down and identify the following:

- Data to be acquired
- Records needed
- Statements received from involved personnel (any out?)
- Instruction manuals, policies, literature, etc.
- Personnel to interview, and
- Additional RCA team members (if desired)

### *The team's first responsibility: Have a meeting*

As soon as possible, the team needs to gather for its first meeting. A good way to begin the first discussion with team members is to explain that the purpose of the investigation is to find fact—not fault—with the individuals involved in the event.

## Begin the investigation

As stated, the purpose of the investigation is to find fact, not fault. Direct the focus of the analysis toward the systems and processes that could have contributed to the event. You might even put people at ease by presenting an example of an RCA in which it appeared at first that specific persons were at fault, but in the end it was demonstrated that a series of system failures were the cause.

### *Debrief the people involved*

(*See the Appendix for a sample form for debriefing purposes*)
Some key questions for the root cause analyst to review prior to debriefing the individuals involved include the following:

*What?*
   — What equipment, person, or tool?
   — What is wrong? What is the complaint?
   — What undesired behavior is involved?

*Who?*

— Which individuals are involved? (Employees? Patients? Staff? Suppliers? Bystanders?)

*When?*

— When did the incident occur (day, date, time)?

— What shift or phase of operation?

— During what part of the plant/equipment life cycle?

— What time pattern is involved?

*Where?*

— What unit, area, or department?

— Where is the defective item or defect on item located?

*How?*

— How is the "what" or "who" affected? (Injury? Death? Patient Injury?)

— How is safety or the environment affected?

— How is the normal conduct of business affected?

### Describe the situation before, during, and after the incident

This step should take place as soon as possible after the incident occurs. During the observation, take photographs (if at all possible) or sketch equipment, the facility, or the process layout to communicate the processes involved.

Carefully document the time and date of each photograph and label it. Insert photos and sketches after this page.

Also, note the work environment conditions at the time of the event. Was it crowded? Noisy? Cluttered? Were there outside influences that were out of the ordinary? Is it before or after a holiday or vacation? What day of the week is it? Were employees working overtime or working after a change in shift?

Don't worry if you think that this is not applicable—sometimes you can glean valuable data from what appears to be extraneous information.

### Conduct interviews

Interviewing can be the most useful tool in data collection. Interviewing is a skill that is developed over time and can be time consuming, but it provides first-hand information and insight into behavior involved in an event. Note that the longer the time interval between the incident and the interview, the less effective interviews become.

There are two phases for interviewing:

1. The initial interview
2. Follow-up interviews

See the Appendix for more information about how to conduct effective interviews.

### Interviewing: Initial

How to conduct an interview (check each step when completed)

### 1) Prepare and plan the interview

❏ Prepare sufficient copies of an initial interview form.

❏ Allow time between interviews to reconstruct notes.

❏ Establish a neutral physical setting, considering privacy and the possibility of interruptions. Consider a closed room (not your office) where an employee can talk freely without worrying about being overheard.

### 2) Open the interview

❏ Put the interviewee at ease. Maintain eye contact, use good vocal expression, and smile.

❏ Exchange small talk. Begin with a sincere compliment or a question to learn more about the interviewee. You may want to establish a common ground based on work experience.

❏ State the purpose of the interview. Indicate why you are conducting the interview and why you are talking to the interviewee.

❏ Say to the interviewee:

• "I wanted to talk to you because . . . "

• "The information we discuss will be combined with other interviews and included in a report to describe the . . . incident."

• "Your name will not be used. All comments will remain anonymous."

• "The interview should take about an hour."

• "Do you have any questions about the process?"

❏ Set the ground rules—let the interviewee know you will be asking questions directly from the form and will not discuss any of the questions or the answers during the initial interview. Explain that you'll interview all interviewees using the same rules.

### 3) Conduct the interview

❏ Listen carefully to the responses and take detailed and exact notes. Do not be afraid to ask the interviewee to slow down or to repeat a statement.

❏ Don't hesitate to take notes on physical and emotional reactions of the interviewee (fidgety, nervous, friendly, open, angry, afraid, upset, sad, confused).

### 4) Conclude the interview

❏ Thank the interviewee (sincerely) for his or her time and cooperation.

❏ Indicate that a follow-up interview may be necessary.

❏ As soon as the interview is over, rewrite your notes so they can be read and understood by others.

**IMPORTANT: At this point, you should be analyzing data. You should use an event and causal factor chart to focus additional data collection. See the Appendix for more information about event and causal factor charting.**

Don't jump to conclusions at this point in the investigation. You will begin to understand possible causes of the incident. Consider all options before declaring the root cause. A common pitfall is to believe an incident was the result of some particular event, which compromises your investigation.

### Interviewing: follow-up

It is very important to conduct initial interviews using the questionnaire in Step 4 before any follow-up interviews. Follow-up interviews must be carefully planned, and are not as standard as the initial format. Questions should be focused, but not leading. Leading questions put words into the interviewee's mouth or unintentionally tell the interviewee how to respond. Follow-up interviews may involve "custom questions." Ask open-ended questions so you may follow-up on answers from the initial discussion, But you do not want to accuse them of not giving you enough information during the first interview. Some traps to avoid in a follow-up interview include the following:

- Asking questions that dictate the answer
- Asking questions that put the interviewee on the defensive
- Asking questions that are too narrowly focused (you don't get the entire story)

The following are some examples of ways to preface questions you may want to ask:
- When we talked before you said . . .
- Can you help me understand . . .
- What did you mean by . . .
- Tell me more about . . .

During your follow-up interviews, remember to record the name of the interviewee, and the questions, and to use the techniques from the initial interviews. Record answers word-for-word.

The purpose of follow-up interviews is to obtain missing information.

Once you complete the interviews, the team can begin to focus on its analysis of the information collected to date.

### *Determine the sequence of events*

Using the information collected so far, establish a timeline of activities leading up to the event. Start with the event and work backward. Identify all pertinent information, including changes of people, procedures, etc. and the environment surrounding each point in time. Be factual without passing judgments ("just the facts, ma'am"). Qualify, validate, and verify (QV&V™) the information. Nothing can discredit later conclusions more quickly than when someone points out, "But that's not how it really happened."

One of the most effective tools to use is the Event & Causal Factor (ECF) charting technique. (See the Appendix for details about developing ECF charts.)

Start by generating a sequence of events. In the event of an injection of potassium chloride, the sequence might cover only several hours, while in the case of an inpatient suicide it might be months. If possible, develop the ECF chart on the computer, using a projector on the screen so that it can be easily seen and modified. During this time, people will start suggesting causes, solutions, etc. Write them down in the parking lot, avoiding discussion of anything but the event sequence for now. Make the sequence detailed and complete, and continue until everyone is satisfied. This will typically take about one hour. Save it to disk.

Have the team look at the sequence and mark every item that might have contributed. Brainstorm and let the group come up with any and all ideas about events, conditions, or anything that might in some way have contributed to (not caused) the adverse event. Use the "parking lot" method to record ideas that are solutions or incidental-but-interesting thoughts that may yield other opportunities for performance improvement. This allows you to postpone these other subjects to another time.

You may identify areas of insufficient data, or you may be able to place new items at other levels. Your goal is to go as far as possible with the facilitator and team leader asking the question, "Why?" until it can no longer be meaningfully asked or answered. (This is called "drill down.") Code each of the bottom items of every branch as "Insufficient Data," "Noncontributory," or "Contributory."

### Construct an initial event chart

**Note:** Begin charting the incident as soon as possible.

An incident is composed of many separate events. An event is an action or happening that occurs during some activity. To begin developing the initial event chart, record the initial event (or earliest related event or beginning point) on a sticky note and the terminal event (or ending point) on a separate sticky note. An event requires an action word (a verb). Each event should begin with an action word and has an associated the date and time. See the example below:

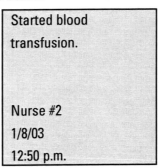

Started blood
transfusion.


Nurse #2
1/8/03
12:50 p.m.

Continue filling out sticky notes until all events contributing to the incident are displayed chronologically from left to right, as illustrated on the next page.

| Received low-level alarm. | Energized bypass machine. | Noticed burning smell. |
|---|---|---|
| Nurse #3<br>1/8/03<br>12:40 p.m. | Technician #2<br>1/8/03<br>12:50 p.m. | Physician #2<br>1/8/03<br>12:55 p.m. |

Arrange and rearrange the notes until you have them in the correct order from the start to the end of the event. This chart will be updated, assessed, and reassessed until all available data have been discovered and included. This chart will form the backbone of the final event and factor chart.

### Determine internal drivers of human error

Use basic RCA tools (see samples in the Appendix) to help identify human errors and inappropriate actions:

- — Structured interviews
- — ECF charts
- — Change analysis
- — Barrier analysis
- — Task analysis
- — Stream analysis
- — RCA tool selection matrix

**Note:** The matrix provided in the Appendix displays a quick reference to the basic RCA tools included in this text and the types of issues each is most effective in analyzing.

Expand the ECF chart by identifying Inappropriate Actions (IAs). A change analysis or barrier analysis may be used to identify relevant circumstances surrounding each of the IAs.

Each IA should have only one subject and one action (i.e., "Doctor X performed an undersized repair" is a clear IA). "Nurse Y missed the pinch clamp on the IV line" is another clear IA. However, "Pinch clamp found on IV line" is a vague IA, because it has no subject but at least one IA.

For each IA, determine the immediate internal factors that caused it. The investigator should identify the following human error factors with the appropriate techniques:

- Human error types—skill/rule/knowledge-based (See Chapter 11 for more information.)
- Human error/IA failure modes (Turn to the Appendix for a chart that lists all human error/IA failure modes.) Identify internal failure modes and the results of interviews with those individuals involved. Update the E&CF chart.

**Note:** The investigator may have to interview the involved person(s) again to confirm the determination.

### *Assess the extent of condition (impact of the evidenced failure)*

In addition to assessing the impact of the immediate failure analyzed an RCA, you must also consider the extent of the failure. In other words, now that symptoms of the failure that triggered the reason for our root cause have been identified, where else might these same symptoms cause a problem that has not yet been discovered? This type of review is also referred to as a "transportability" review. Where else could we reasonably expect to "transport" the failure mode and be subject to the same deficiencies?

For example, if an autoclave is found to be faulty and does not provide adequate time or temperature for complete removal of bacteria, actions to correct this problem would include replacing or repairing the sterilizer, resterilizing instruments not effectively cleaned in the compromised batch, and performing a failure analysis to determine the cause for the failure and actions to prevent recurrence for this equipment. However, long before the root cause of the equipment failure is determined, the impact of the symptoms observed (sterilizer that does not achieve adequate time/temperature to provide adequate sanitation) must be assessed. This is called the "extent of condition" or the extent to which the identified symptoms can cause a problem.

In order to determine the extent of condition for this example, you need to determine the following:

1. The number of other potentially contaminated instruments are out there, having been cleaned with this same piece of equipment
2. How many other sterilizers do we have that could potentially demonstrate this same failure mode?

Actions to address the extent of condition might include the following:

- A determination of the most recent point at which the sterilizer was known to function properly (after which point it is reasonable to suspect cleanliness of anything cleaned by it)
- A review all instruments cleaned with the faulty machine from the date it was last determined to be operational
- A review of all other sterilizers that are found to be subject to the same failure mode

The review to determine the "extent" of the potential failure must be done as soon as observed symptoms are known and the impact of these symptoms is understood well enough to ask appropriate "extent of condition or transportability" questions.

Later, after the cause of the failure has been determined we will ask other transportability" questions related to the potential for the root cause(s) identified to drive other failures. This potential is referred to as the generic implication of the cause(s) or transportability of the cause.

## Summary

At this point in the RCA process, you have completed Step 1 in the RCA process. However, you will find that although we will move on to the next step—collecting information and data—RCA often involves jumping back to steps previously performed to repeat actions as new information becomes available. So keep the actions of Step 1 in mind as you move on to the next chapter.

In the next chapter we will discuss specific types of information and data that will be needed to support your analysis and the most effective means of collection.

# CHAPTER 4

## Just the Facts, Please!
## Collecting Data and Information

# CHAPTER 4

---

# Just the Facts, Please!
# Collecting Data and Information

## STEP 2

## Overview—before you begin . . . read on

It is very likely that you will not be able to answer the questions posed to you in Chapter 3 regarding transportability (or applicability) of the event of interest without collecting some very specific information and data. In this chapter we'll discuss particular lessons learned that can make this aspect of your work much more focused and efficient.

## Data collection

Data you'll need to collect include the following:
- Physical evidence
- Documents
- History of past events or similar incidents

To be able to adequately meet the standards for "thorough and credible" you'll need to collect all available data to help determine when, where, why, and how the incident occurred, and who was involved. Data collection should include information about conditions before, during, and after the event. Collect and review information in the following areas:

- **Observations** (including actions taken) of personnel who were involved in or witnessed the event, through direct interview and written statements. In general, conduct initial interviews and written statements within 24 hours; however, subsequent follow-up interviews may be held during the early weeks of the investigation. (A recommended format for written statements is provided in the Appendix.)

---

- Note and log defective materials or equipment (supplies, monitors, intravenous or bypass pumps, etc) or at a minimum, keep photographs of the problem areas. Include patient charts, or photocopies of pertinent areas of the chart.

- Use representative samples of consumable supplies for later analysis and simulation.

- Record environmental factors and any special conditions present.

- Document accounts of any activities related to the event or condition (develop layout sketches as necessary).

- Review similar events that occurred in the past. (In most cases, a 2-year period is enough to satisfy the standards of "thorough and credible." We'll talk more about this later in the chapter.)

- Know human performance or medical procedure issues associated with the event.

- Research recent program or personnel changes.

- Collect data as soon after the incident as possible. Delays in data collection allow people to recall the situation differently than it actually occurred.

### *Tips for collecting data*

Keep the following in mind when collecting data:

1. Collect data in a timely manner.
2. Use basic methods for recording information (written, recorded, pictorial).
3. Properly identify and log the source, date and time, location, basic content and purpose, and name of the person making the record.
4. Take complete notes to ensure accuracy and completeness and to facilitate report preparation. Well-taken and complete notes are a valuable historical reference. All notes should be organized and dated.

Some key questions to ask when collecting data include the following:

*What?*

       — What is wrong? What is the complaint?

       — What equipment, monitoring devices, instruments, supplies?

       — What undesired behavior?

Who?

— Who was involved? (Staff? Physicians? Technicians? Pharmacy? Management?)

When?

— When did the incident occur? (day, date, time)

— During what shift or phase of rotation?

— What time pattern is involved?

Where?

— What unit, department, or area?

— Connected to main facility or not?

— Separated geographically from facility?

— Where is the defective item or defect on an item located?

How?

— What or who has been affected? (Injury? Death? Type or classification?)

— What about patient's health or safety and to whom?

— How is safety or the environment affected?

— How is operation of the facility affected?

— How are finances affected?

— How many affected individuals (patients or employees)?

— How many times was patient affected?

### Collect, document, label, and preserve all physical evidence

Make sure that you collect all physical evidence related to the event. Physical evidence can include any of the following:

- Failed instruments
- Ruptured bags
- Burned leads
- Blown fuses
- Spilled body or chemical fluids
- Broken syringes
- Partially completed work orders or procedures

## Information from interviews

In Chapter 3, we dedicated considerable time and space to the preparation and conduct of interviews to collect important information.

At this point in the investigative process, the majority of interviewing is done. However, there may be additional information that is needed to be able to "rule in or rule out" a particular failure possibility. If this is the case, you will need to conduct follow-up interviews.

The information from follow-up interviews is often needed to qualify, validate, and independently verify information into facts that can be used to support or refute potential causes of the event. Once interviews are done, the team can focus on its analysis of the information collected to date.

## Qualification, validation, and verification (QV&V) of raw information into facts

### *What is QV&V?*

QV&V is a technique to ensure decisions you make rely on factual information and data. QV&V is also referred to as a "questioning attitude" technique.

Questioning attitude involves performing the following checks on information that will be used in making decisions throughout the investigation:

**Step 1: Qualification**—Check the information source to be sure it is reliable
**Step 2: Validation**—Check the information to be sure it "makes sense to me"
**Step 3: Verification**—Use an independent source to corroborate

### *How do I perform QV&V?*

- Most people already perform steps one and two (above); these steps are very typical in human nature. We are always making judgments about what we see, hear, and are subjected to. When we compare those judgments with our own personal experiences and knowledge, we are actually doing the "validation" step in QV&V.

- Generally what will get you into trouble is having a gut feeling as you look at validating information or direction we get from others; that it is wrong or somehow incomplete and we don't follow up on that feeling.

- Most people won't perform step #3 unless they are certain there is a problem. The verification step—checking with an independent source—is a critical success factor for determining the real strength of information we might use to perform a task.

Let's look at each step in a little more detail.

## Step 1: Qualify

**Qualification** considers the information source, not the information. Relevant details are not omitted.

Ask yourself these questions:
- Is this information relevant to my problem or decision?
- Am I getting this information from a source that I consider reliable and truthful?
- Do I have any reason to suspect anything but high quality from the source?

Information should always come from a source commensurate with the risk associated with an error (the higher the risk, the more critical the source). Good sources of information include consensus standards, protocols, and written data prepared in accordance with procedures. Lesser sources of information include oral communications, informal written communications, and uncorroborated opinion.

Often you will go to "easy" sources of information that may not be up to date or accurate (i.e., going to someone who used to be the guru in a certain area and soliciting information because they are available, rather than going to the person who now has responsibility). It is best to go back to the original source of the data/information, since other individuals are often unclear or inaccurate about information/instructions and end up reinforcing or adding bad information.

## Step 2: Validate

**Validation** is an internal examination of the information. In validation, you'll compare the information to what is already known. This is a consistency check.

You do not need to ensure that the information is correct, but must at least ensure that the information is consistent with what they know as fact and would expect to be fact. Validation ensures that all of the user's knowledge and skill are consciously applied to select the course of action.

## Step 3: Verify

**Verification** is an external check. This step is performed by finding an independent and qualified source to corroborate the rule or information. The emphasis is on "independent."

A second qualified person is the least-preferred source because people in organizations tend to share the same bad information. Documents, physical evidence, and diverse instrumentation are always more reliable sources for verification.

Many independent sources are available to verify information we use in decision-making. For example, when driving, a map may be the tool most often used to verify accurate driving instructions.

### Use QV&V to turn raw information into facts that can be used to support or refute your cause analysis

Keep a list of the information that you believe will be important in making a determination of the root and contributing causes in the investigation. This list, usually kept in table format or a spreadsheet (for easier sorting by keywords), drives the collection of information from follow-up interviews and evidence analysis that will be needed to provide factual results to support the conclusions of your investigation.

Once you establish what information you have, you determine what is needed to qualify, validate, and verify key pieces of information so you can consider them factual and therefore good enough to use in your "supporting and refuting" activities.

It is very important to take this step so you don't jump to conclusions at this point of the investigation. You will be starting to understand possible causes for the incident. Be careful to consider all the options using the techniques to support or refute each possible cause (found in the next chapter) prior to declaring the root cause and claiming victory.

A common pitfall at this point in the process is to form a personal belief early on that an incident was the result of a particular event and not use the supporting and refuting analysis to confirm or deny that belief. This compromises your investigation and may ultimately result in very ineffective corrective actions.

## Frequently asked questions and answers

Before we leave the topic of information and data, there are two questions that come up routinely in our work that we'd like to address.

1) Can software be used to expedite the process?
2) Why must we look at past history and literature as a part of the process?

### Does software help in root cause analysis?

At about this time in an investigation, analysts are buried in information and data, and are asked, "Can software can help with an RCA?" The answer is yes and no.

### The first answer is yes

We have found the use of software products that boost the efficiency and effectiveness with which individual "tasks" can be accomplished within the RCA to be very valuable. For example, data logging, manipulation and control programs (e.g., Microsoft Access, Microsoft Excel, etc.) are very helpful in keeping track of and processing large amounts of data.

### The second answer is no

We have seen more than we'd like to see of overworked analysts who drive the review of an event from their desks, never setting foot near the location of the event, the individuals involved in the event, and in some cases, even the state of the event. They collect just the minimum information necessary to get through a "branch" of a decision tree in the software, attributing the cause of the investigation to the first likely candidate that sounds defensible. So, instead of the analysis of information and facts driving the selection of codes to reflect root causes in the trending system, the opposite is true. Codes and categories drive the minimum level of effort needed to "justify" their selection and use. Corrective actions "automatically" generated by the computer, based on the results of the decision tree, are not effective. Therefore events are repeated, which drives more events, and the increased use of the software.

### Why must we look at past history and literature as a part of the process?

The following are the four basic reasons that dictate performance of appropriate reviews of pertinent literature as part of your RCA:

1. Identify standards of care, or other standards that have application to the adverse event or circumstance under analysis.
2. Benefit from lessons learned by other health care organizations in similar circumstances.
3. Identify alternative corrective actions or practices that have been published elsewhere.
4. Convince the Joint Commission on Accreditation of Healthcare Organizations (JCAHO) that you have done the above, to increase the confidence that your RCA has been "thorough and credible."

## Summary

At this point in the process, you have collected and analyzed information and data that will be used to support or refute potential failure modes, also referred to as failure mechanisms, for the event. In the next chapter we'll take you through the process of narrowing this list.

# CHAPTER 5

## How to Identify the Failure Modes

# CHAPTER 5

## How to Identify the Failure Modes

**STEP 3**

This chapter examines the critical link between identifying the failure modes and discovering the true causes of an adverse event.

So far we've covered the first two steps in the six-step root cause analysis (RCA) process (see Figure 2.2 in Chapter 2) and have accomplished the following:

1. Investigated the adverse incident using basic RCA techniques (i.e., events and causal factor charting) to identify problem statements contributing to the event
2. Determined facts by using data collection and the QV&V technique

The next step is identifying the failure modes (mechanisms) that led to the event by diagnosing the failure mode for each problem statement (Step 1) based on the facts in the case (Step 2). Failure modes are also called primary effects and can occur in the following three ways:

- Equipment failures
- Inappropriate actions
- Externals events

## Equipment failures

Equipment failures and malfunctions are relatively common, contributing to 10% of all patient safety occurrences or events, according to a PII study of 186 health care cases from 2001–2002.

For example, a blanket heater malfunctioned at one hospital and put full heating power into the circulating water. The excess heat caused the water tubing to fail, resulting in second- and third-degree burns to an unconscious ICU patient. At another hospital, an infusion pump malfunctioned, and caused a dramatic increase in the infusion rate, resulting in a narcotics overdose to the patient. Fortunately, the patient survived without any permanent injury thanks to the quick-thinking actions of the primary nurse.

## Inappropriate actions

Inappropriate actions or human errors contribute to approximately 90% of all medical errors (according to the same study of 186 health care cases) and have a well-recognized adverse effect on patient safety. Inappropriate actions that result in harm can happen to any and all professional groups within health care: physicians, nurses, pharmacists, admitting clerks, and even dietary, facility maintenance, and housekeeping personnel. Examples of inappropriate acts range from highly publicized errors, such as a surgeon who amputates a patient's wrong leg, to common errors, such as a nurse who gives a patient the wrong medication.

## External events

External events that cause patient harm are rare. These events include odd happenings, such as a car accidentally driven into a hospital emergency department, causing injury to people in the waiting room. Natural disasters, such as hurricanes, tornadoes, lighting, or earthquakes, would also fall into this category. Unfortunately, another potential type of external event must be added to these: terrorism. Whether it is bioterrorism, such as a small pox attack, or other forms of terrorist-inflicted damage, this is a grim reality of which we must be aware and for which we must prepare our institutions and ourselves.

Hospitals should prepare for the possibility that an external event could act as a primary effect. But, so far in the history of patient safety, external events haven't been significant contributors to patient harm.

Therefore, RCA for patient safety is a matter of diagnosing the causes of equipment failures in a few instances and inappropriate actions in most cases.

## Identifying possible causes

Human error is a manifestation of system problems (refer to the introduction for the Swiss cheese and Sharp-End models). Based on 10 years of RCA for events in complex systems (1,118 cases), PII has found that only 15% of events have an isolated cause—the trigger in the Swiss cheese model. Eighty-five percent have a shared cause in the system—the holes in the Swiss cheese model.

System problems cause most patient safety events due to inappropriate actions (human errors) and equipment failures. Therefore, to improve patient safety you must improve human and equipment performance. To improve human and equipment performance you must improve system performance. Whether you are dealing with a human problem or equipment problem, the first step in solving it is to identify the failure mode.

All RCA techniques accomplish two basic effects: First, they help identify all the possible causes or failure modes; second, they help identify which failure modes are consistent with the facts in the case.

The following are the three basic options to identify all the possible causes:

- Use your own experience if you are an expert
- Consult with experts
- Use diagnostic tools

Experts have vast experience in diagnosing and correcting specific problems, such as human error or the effects of professional standards changes on human error. Experts have seen all failure modes, know the symptoms of each one, and understand the actions needed to correct each failure mode. Unfortunately, most of you performing RCAs are not experts in all of the failures that you would expect to see.

Therefore, most root cause analysts tend to consult with experts to identify a more complete set of all possible failure modes. The problem with this type of consultation is that it takes time, which is a precious commodity for most RCA teams. Experts are also biased by their knowledge—they tend to only think of possible failure modes in their own specialty.

## Diagnostic tools

An RCA team can avoid these problems by using technology-based diagnostic tools to identify all possible causes that led to an adverse event. "Technology-based" means that the tool was developed through a scientific study of cause-and-effect relations. Therefore, there is less risk that the tool has left out a cause, mixed similar causes together, or included possible causes that have no proven cause-and-effect relationship.

Most diagnostic tools are based on limited case experience, not technology. We don't recommend them because they tend to be overly detailed in some areas, vague in others, and rely heavily on the "usual suspects" as possible causes, such as the following:

- Policy and procedure are less than adequate (recommendation is to change the policy)
- Training is less than adequate (recommendation is to get more training)
- Individual performance error is to blame (recommendation is to coach employees not to do it again)

These causes are all conditions in a system. This approach links a condition (as a causal factor) to an adverse event. The theory is that if you remove the condition, you'll prevent the occurrence.

### Failure mode approach

Your RCA team will achieve better results by using a failure mode approach. Failure modes are ways that systems fail (refer to Chapter 11 for a detailed explanation of the term). In this approach, root cause analysts or teams link the occurrence to a primary effect (an inappropriate action or an equipment failure). First, they identify the failure mode of the primary effect. Then they study the conditions that combined to form the failure mode. The theory with this approach is that if you remove the substandard condition forming the failure mode, you will prevent recurrence of the primary effect and the event.

This approach is best illustrated on a failure mode diagram, which is a graphical depiction of all possible failure modes of a specific primary effect (see Figure 5.1).

The diagram is simple to use. The primary effect is shown at the top. All the possible failure modes are depicted in the text boxes. Failure mode diagrams have two critical traits: the failure modes are mutually exclusive and collectively exhaustive (MECE).

Mutually exclusive means the primary effect (failure) cannot be the result of a combination of failure modes. The phrase, "comprehensively exhaustive," means that the analysis includes all known possible failure modes.

Figure 5.2 is an example failure mode diagram for a very simple piece of medical equipment: an orthopedic screw used in a surgical procedure to join bones.

The screw is well thought out in design, manufacture, and in application to prevent failure. But a screw can fail in a finite and known number of ways (or modes), including the following:
- overload
- fatigue
- shear-out of the base material
- corrosion
- embrittlement

**Figure 5.1** "Failure Mode Diagram"

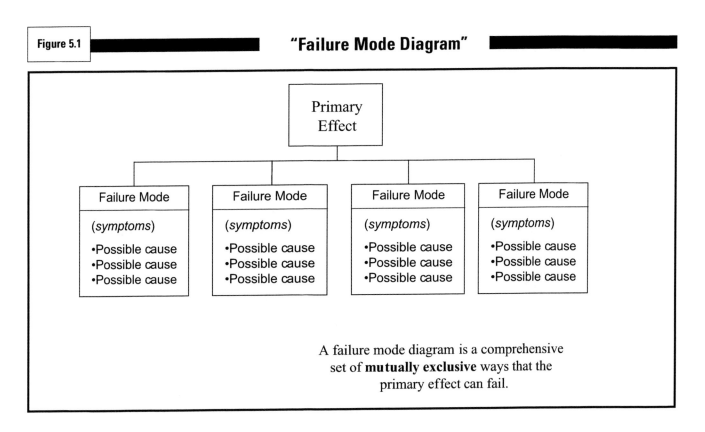

A failure mode diagram is a comprehensive set of **mutually exclusive** ways that the primary effect can fail.

**Figure 5.2** Example Failure Mode Diagram for Orthopedic Screw Failure

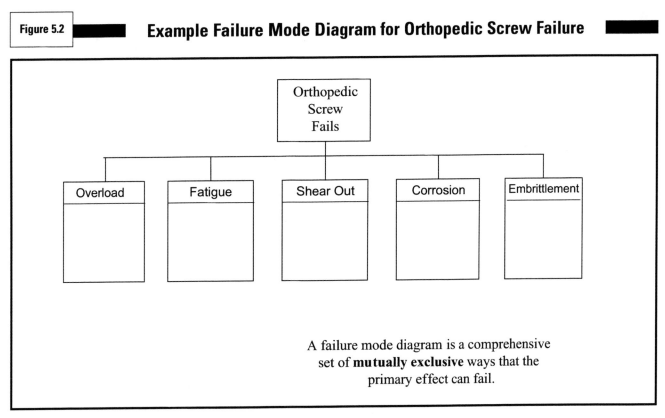

A failure mode diagram is a comprehensive set of **mutually exclusive** ways that the primary effect can fail.

If the diagram for the screw really is MECE, the failure mode explaining the primary effect (screw breaks) must be one of those boxes on the diagram. Which box is it? The true failure mode is the one that is consistent with all the facts in the case. It is supported by some facts in the case and refuted by none. (Some facts in the case may neither support nor refute a failure mode.) And the facts in the case refute all other possible failure modes.

To use a failure mode diagram, list all facts in the case that are related to the primary effect. Consider each fact as it relates to a possible failure mode. If the fact is consistent with the failure mode, the condition is known to exist when the failure mode is present, then the fact supports the failure mode. If the fact is inconsistent with the failure mode (it doesn't exist when the mode is present), the fact refutes the failure mode.

This approach allows you to eliminate failure modes with refuting facts. The team continues using this support/refute method until only one failure mode remains. The remaining one is the true failure for the primary effect in the case.

What happens if this approach eliminates all possible failure modes? Either the failure mode diagram was incomplete and didn't include one or two failure modes or the team eliminated a failure mode based on an incorrect fact. To avoid this problem, check to make sure the failure mode diagram is complete and double-check the facts in the case.

### The evidence matrix

A quick and simple method to support or refute possible failure modes is through an evidence matrix or table (see Figure 5.3). The table shows each possible failure mode, the supporting facts, and the refuting facts.

Root cause analysts often use the evidence matrix when establishing a failure mode that is critical to the case, especially equipment or medical device failures that result in legal action. They usually don't use it for inappropriate actions. Instead, most analysts present the facts in the case and offer the failure mode that is consistent with those facts. A very obscure or complicated inappropriate action is a notable exception.

### Human error failure modes

Inappropriate actions trigger most patient safety occurrences. People are definitely more complicated than orthopedic screws. Although there are billions of people on the planet, each with an individual personality, talents, and flaws, there are only 28 possible human error failure modes that we all share. These failure modes include the following:

| Figure 5.3 | **Evidence Matrix (to support and refute each mode)** |

| Failure Mode | Supporting Facts | Refuting Facts | Actions to Complete |
|---|---|---|---|
| Overload | Ductile failure region on 40% of fracture surface | Breach marks (or crack arrest lines) on 40% of fracture surface. | None |
| Fatigue | Breach marks (or crack arrest lines) on 40% of fracture surface. | | Estimate stress and endurance limit of screw. |

**Attention-related modes:**

1. Unawareness
2. Pressure to complete task
3. Task complexity
4. Job distractions

**Misjudgment-related modes:**

5. Cognitive overload
6. Habit intrusion
7. Spatial misorientation
8. Mindset
9. Wrong assumptions
10. Lack of validation and verification
11. Misinterpretation

**Committed actions, not performed modes:**

12. Shortcuts evoked

13. Task complexity

14. Inappropriate orders

15. Job distractions

16. Inadequate mental tracking

**Inadequate skills or knowledge modes:**

17. Tunnel vision

18. Inadequate skill development

19. Not familiar with job standards

20. Not familiar with task

21. Not familiar with availability of information

**Inadequate mental state modes:**

22. Boredom

23. Lapse of memory

24. Reflex

25. Fear of failure

26. Illness, fatigue, injury, or sickness

27. Overconfidence

28. Inadequate motivation

Displayed as a diagnostic chart, a failure mode diagram for human error/inappropriate actions is shown in Figure 5.4.

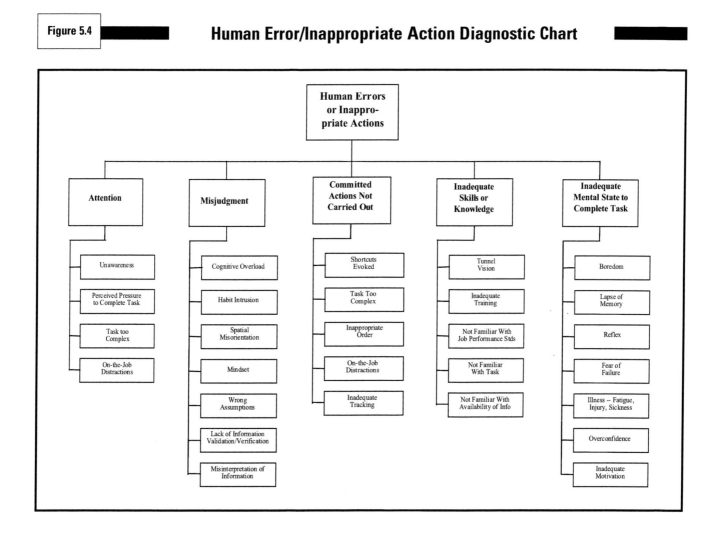

Figure 5.4 — Human Error/Inappropriate Action Diagnostic Chart

Use this diagnostic tool just as you would in Figure 5.2, the failure mode diagram for the orthopedic screw. This chart shows all of the possible failure modes for people. Use facts in the case to rule out failure modes until you are left with one that is consistent with all the facts in the case.

## Questions to consider

*Can there be more than one failure mode for an inappropriate action?*

No. Each failure mode is mutually exclusive so there is a one-to-one correspondence between inappropriate action and the human error failure mode. If two failure modes are apparent(especially two radically different ones) present, look for two inappropriate actions occurring closely together.

For example, the first inappropriate action is an incorrect improvisation. A person deviates from the process (an improvisation), and takes a different action (the second inappropriate action) that is unsuccessful. This results in two inappropriate actions, each with a single failure mode. There is also the corresponding case of the correct improvisation. The person deviates from the process (an inappropriate action), but takes an action that is successful. In this instance, the result is only one inappropriate act with one failure mode.

A health care example of an incorrect improvisation occurs when a nurse misidentifies a patient as part of the medication administration process. The process, as it was designed, requires the nurse to bring the medication administration record (MAR) into the patient's room to compare name and date of birth to the patient's identification bracelet. A nurse may leave the MAR in the medication room (the improvisation) and then compounds the problem by confusing this patient's name with another. Two inappropriate actions take place, each with a single failure mode.

## The health care system

Similarly, there are finite and known sets of failure modes for work environment (14 modes), human factors (14 modes), human error (28 modes) organizations and processes (18 modes), and management (30 modes).  (See the Appendix for charts on each set of failure modes.) Together, these failure mode systems comprise all the ways a health care system can fail.

Remember that the intent of Step 3 in the six-step RCA process is to determine a failure mode for each problem statement (primary effect) in the occurrence. In addition, primary effects can be equipment failures or external events, but are usually inappropriate actions.

Although inappropriate actions and equipment failures shape patient safety occurrences, the health care delivery system shapes the inappropriate actions and equipment failures. The idea in performing RCA is very simple:

- Start with the outcome (occurrence)
- Identify inappropriate actions (or equipment failures) that led to the outcome
- Determine the failure mode for each inappropriate action (or equipment failures)
- Determine the system failure modes that shape the inappropriate actions (or equipment failures)

The health care system is shown in Figure 5.5.

Inappropriate actions by people and medical equipment and device failures are the proximate causes of patient harm. But we should not blame the people who commit inappropriate actions. Instead, we must recognize that the system shapes human behavior. Human factors and the design of equipment and med-

Figure 5.5 ██████████ **"The Healthcare Delivery System"** ██████████

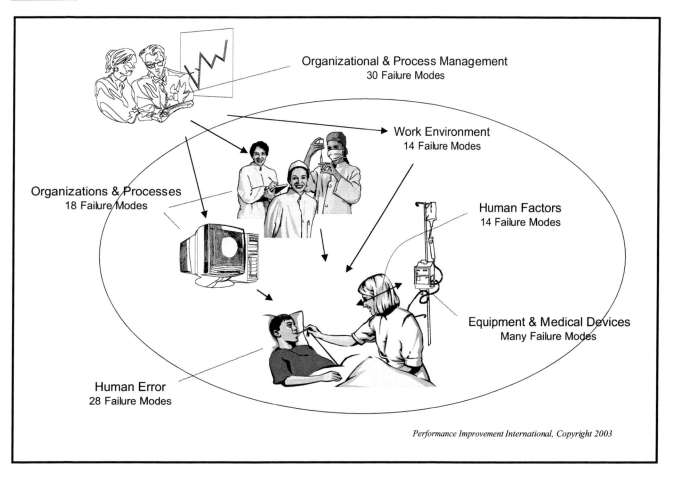

Organizational & Process Management
30 Failure Modes

Work Environment
14 Failure Modes

Organizations & Processes
18 Failure Modes

Human Factors
14 Failure Modes

Equipment & Medical Devices
Many Failure Modes

Human Error
28 Failure Modes

*Performance Improvement International, Copyright 2003*

ical devices can increase the probability of human error. Work environment factors such as lighting and noise, or task factors such as workload and multi-tasking, also can increase human error rate.

People do not work alone. People work in organizations, and organizational effects can have strong negative effects on human error rate. People also work according to policy and procedure (the work process). Focused and simplified processes have strong positive effects on human error rate; complex and fragmented processes have negative effects. Hospital leaders (nurse managers, pharmacy directors, vice presidents of medical affairs, etc.) must care for the organizations, processes, and work environment much like nurses care for patients.

In this approach, there is a clear link between the system failure that shaped the inappropriate action(s) and the inappropriate action(s) that harmed the patient.

## Summary

This chapter explained the importance of using technology-based diagnostic tools to identify all the possible failure modes and how to pinpoint the failure mode for each inappropriate action or equipment failure using supporting/refuting facts. In the next chapter (**Chapter 6,** Develop the Failure Scenario[s]), we will discuss how to determine system failure modes related to inappropriate actions and equipment failures.

# CHAPTER 6

## Develop the Failure Scenario(s)

# CHAPTER 6

---

# Develop the Failure Scenario(s)

**STEP 4**

Developing the failure scenario is Step 4 in the six-step root cause analysis (RCA) process. At this point in the process, you've performed Steps 1–3 and accomplished the following:

1. Investigated the occurrence using basic RCA techniques (event and causal-factor charting) to identify problem statements contributing to the occurrence

2. Determined facts by using data collection and the QV&V technique

3. identified the failure modes for each primary effect: inappropriate action, equipment failure, or medical device failure

The failure scenario is a narrative story that begins with the root cause(s) and proceeds through the failure mode(s) and primary effect(s) to the event. Failure scenarios are always constructed backward because of information availability. A root cause analyst's first piece of information is the consequence associated with the sentinel event. Next, the investigator learns the primary effects (mostly inappropriate actions) followed by the failure mode for each one. Eventually, the investigator or RCA team will discover the conditions in the system that led to the failure modes. At least one of these failure modes will lead to a root cause of the event.

Although we construct failure scenarios in a reverse sequence, the story is best understood when told in chronological order. Start with the root cause(s) and describe the cause-and-effect relationships leading to the consequence observed in the adverse event.

---

Developing the failure scenario is the process of moving from a failure mode to a root cause. We already learned that a failure mode is a unique combination of conditions that form together to result in a specific effect. A root cause is a condition in the system that if corrected or removed prevents recurrence of the event. So in practice, a root cause is a system condition that is a part of or contributes to the unique combination of conditions required for the observed failure mode.

## From failure mode to root cause

Every failure mode is composed of a unique combination of conditions that result in a specific effect. This combination of conditions acts much like a recipe. If you change or substitute one important ingredient, you will get a different result. For example, a cake without baking powder will not rise.

Similarly, if you change one of the conditions that makes up a failure mode, you will get a different effect. Each failure mode has a definite recipe. Taking away one ingredient in the recipe prevents recurrence of the failure mode. Changing the system so that you remove one or more ingredients will prevent recurrence of the failure mode, the primary effect, and the negative occurrence. So in effect, the ingredient removed was the root cause of the adverse event.

### A health care example

Now consider the case of a simple, inappropriate action. A surgeon is scheduled to perform a procedure to correct a patient's left number-two hammer-toe. The patient needs the procedure on both feet, but is having them performed one at a time so that she can care for her infirmed husband. Both feet are prepared and exposed when the surgeon enters the operating room. (The fact that this was the case means other inappropriate actions occurred in the process that led to this point; but this case study focuses just on the surgeon's inappropriate action.) The surgical site identification policy and procedure requires the surgeon to identify the toe by verifying the site mark and confirming laterality with the medical record and consent form. The toe isn't marked and the surgeon chooses not to verify the site with the medical record because this is such a simple procedure. He has been heard to say he knows his patients by name and does not need to doodle on them with a felt-tip marker. In this moment he also knows for a fact that this patient needs both a left and a right number-two hammer-toe repair.

The occurrence in this case is a surgical procedure performed on the wrong site of the right patient. While there are no actual patient safety consequences as the result of this error, the patient will likely be unsatisfied with the result.

Of the 28 human error failure modes (see **Chapter 5**), this example falls under "shortcuts evoked." The surgeon chose not to verify the site though he knew that he should have and thought about it at the time. The failure mode has the following four prerequisites:

1. The person knows the requirement well and is capable (no skill or knowledge problems)
2. The person knows the requirement is applicable to the situation (no misjudgment)
3. The person knows the requirement at the time (no memory lapse or attention problem)
4. The person chooses an alternate action thinking the choice is the same or better

In this case, the surgeon chose not to comply with a requirement of which he was aware. To understand why individuals don't comply with requirements of which they are aware—a remarkably common problem in health care—it is helpful to apply the following noncompliance equation:

$$\text{Noncompliance} = \frac{\text{Perceived burden}}{\text{Risk awareness} + \text{compliance culture}}$$

Perceived burden is an estimate, as seen through the eyes of the individual worker, of how difficult it is to comply with the requirement. Using the example of handwashing to prevent health care–acquired infections, which is a major noncompliance problem, a worker may perceive a high burden to washing their hands if the soap produces skin irritation. This burden can be reduced by providing antiseptic hand lotions, which would then increase compliance. Risk awareness is a measure of the extent to which the worker perceives significant consequences of noncompliance. If a worker believes that the chance of transferring an infection is remote, he or she is less likely to comply. Compliance culture describes the degree to which fellow workers hold each other accountable for complying with the requirement, not just supervisors.

Note the power in the noncompliance equation (see above equation). When perceived burden in performing the act increases, the noncompliance rate rises. When people are aware of the risk—they know bad outcomes tend to happen if they don't do it—the noncompliance rate goes down. If the hospital's patient safety culture improves and most employees comply with proper procedures, those who don't follow policy will feel the effects through peer pressure and their rate of compliance will increase.

In the surgeon's case, there were two elements of the noncompliance equation:

1. The surgeon has low risk awareness for wrong procedure/site/person surgery.
2. The compliance culture in the operating room is weak (the team didn't question the fact that both patient's feet were exposed and everyone on the surgical team allowed the surgeon to proceed with the operation.)

The root cause(s) rest on these two paths. In this case, the solution was primarily through enhancing the compliance culture in the operating room.

### *A health care example*

Consider another example. Two housekeepers stripped the wax from the floor of a magnetic resonance imaging (MRI) suite in radiology. All the tools they used were plastic because the magnet was very powerful and was always on. Special precautions were taken to ensure that there was no metal on or in the housekeepers to avoiding attraction/heating from the intense magnetic field. The hospital ensured that staff take these precautions to protect the workers, the magnet, and the patient undertaking the MRI. (One publicized sentinel event took place at an East Coast hospital in which a young patient was killed when a steel oxygen cylinder struck his head during an MRI study.)

After the housekeepers completed the procedure, they were impatient as they waited for the floor to dry. To speed up the process, one housekeeper went to the shop and returned with a blower. The second housekeeper tried to intercede and they had the following exchange:

"You can't bring that in here."

"Don't worry, it's plastic."

"Oh, . . . well, okay then."

The blower had a plastic case and a plastic fan wheel. However, the motor had a steel frame and shaft and the windings and wiring were copper. The "all plastic" fan flew from the housekeeper's hands across the room and centered itself in the field of the magnet. Fortunately, neither housekeeper suffered an injury, but the magnet was damaged and was out of service for a few days.

The occurrence in this case is a precursor event in MRI safety. There were no actual safety consequences, but there were financial results and probably patient safety issues due to the fact the machine was out of service. The event is significant because of its potential consequences. Had this occurred at another time under slightly different circumstances, it may have resulted in an injury to a patient or health care provider.

There are two inappropriate actions in this example. The first housekeeper brought the fan into the magnet room of the MRI suite. The second housekeeper wasn't thinking clearly and failed to stop him. Consider only the second housekeeper in this case.

Of the 28 human error failure modes, the second housekeeper made a conscious choice to allow the first housekeeper to bring in the blower. This was a misjudgment, specifically lack of validation and verification. The failure mode has the following recipe:

- The person receives incorrect or incomplete information (the blower is plastic)
- The person uses the information in a judgment or decision ("well okay then")
- The person should have known the information was incorrect or incomplete
- The person fails in critical thinking (the common sense meter in the brain fails)

Since the first three ingredients of the recipe are often present in the system, the fourth (critical thinking) is the best path to the root cause. (Studies on information quality in complex systems indicate that 50% of the information that is used as fact is either insufficiently detailed or inaccurate.) In this case, the best solution is providing behavior-based expectations for critical thinking in the form of questioning attitude with QV&V technique (see the glossary in **Chapter 11** for a complete definition of QV&V).

## Conditions in the recipe are failure modes in the system

Think about the big picture. A condition in the system is also a failure mode of the system. Consider Figure 5.5 in **Chapter 5,** "The Health Care Delivery System." We can describe conditions external to the health care provider that result in human error failure modes as

- human factor deficiencies
- work environment deficiencies
- process (policy and procedure) deficiencies
- organizational breakdowns

This thinking gives us the ability to move beyond the inappropriate action and equipment failures where only 15% of root causes exist as isolated occurrences to the system and 85% of root causes are local or global system failures.

The thought process is the same. Use failure mode diagrams that describe the system as the set of all possible causes. Use facts from the case to support or refute each possible cause. The system failure modes are ones that are supported by facts in the case and refuted by none. So if a root cause analyst used an events and causal factor chart (a basic RCA technique for occurrences involving multiple primary effects), the chart would look something like the simplified example shown in Figure 6.1. Note that other inappropriate actions are not shown in the figure.

Figure 6.1 **"Events and Causal Factor Chart"**

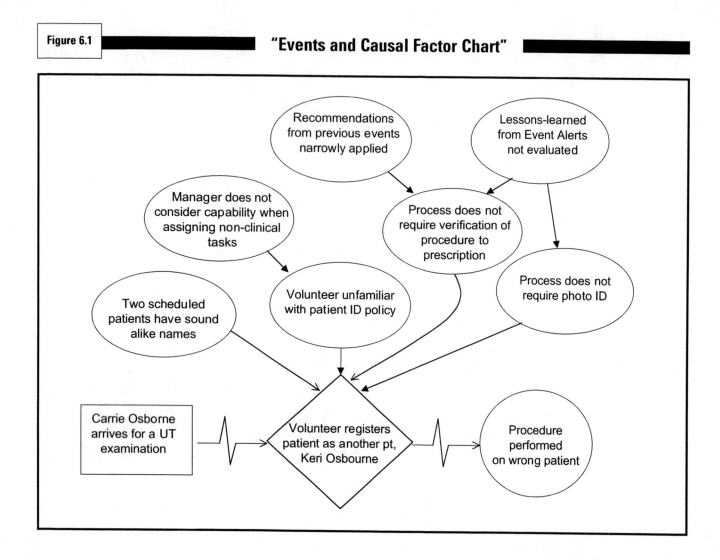

The inappropriate actions are shown in diamond-shaped text boxes. Directly above is the human error failure mode in an oval text box. Above the human error failure mode are the system factors that represent the ingredients of the failure mode recipe. These factors are failure modes of the system.

Each time an RCA team identifies a failure mode, it has asked "why" at least one time. So each level of conditions above a primary effect represents an additional answer. However, the "Five Whys" approach as a rule is not meant to describe how deep he or she should probe into a failure scenario.

The "Five Whys" is an effective and efficient tool for health care providers to use in group problem-solving. However, RCA is not always asking why five times. For some cases it is only asking why two times, and in other cases, eight times. Some cases have multiple primary effects that branch into four root causes with one being somewhat isolated (asked why only two times) and another very deep in the failure scenario (asked why 10 times). Use more structured ideas to identify root causes, especially for patient safety occurrences in which the RCA will in fact be a life-and-death process, one that affects how the health care system will function for the next patient. These ideas must go to two basic ends:

- Knowing what a good root cause condition looks like
- Knowing when to ask "why" again (or at least knowing when to stop asking "why")

## Critical attributes of a root cause

A root cause is a distinct and different condition than a contributing cause. If an RCA team member doesn't know the difference between a root cause and a contributing cause or, worse yet, a normal condition in the system, perhaps he or she shouldn't do a cause analysis. A root cause condition has three critical attributes; that is, three factors that the condition must have to be a root cause. A root cause also has a fourth attribute that is not critical, but is good to have as a confirmation.

First, consider the meaning of "critical attribute," which is a characteristic that absolutely must be present for an item to be specific and unique. Differences in critical attributes distinguish the item from other similar items.

A root cause is a condition in the system that has three critical attributes. The following must be present to verify a root cause:

1. The condition has a proven cause-and-effect relationship. If the hospital removes the condition from the system, it will prevent recurrence and have no harmful side effects.
2. The condition is within management's control to correct.
3. The condition is cost-effective to correct.

A root cause condition also has a fourth attribute that is good to have for confirmation: The condition is substandard.

A contributing cause is a lesser factor than a root cause. Contributing causes are also called exacerbating factors or aggravating factors. They have proven cause-and-effect relationships that make the occurrence worse, but correcting them wouldn't necessarily prevent recurrence.

Since the root cause analyst's job is to prevent recurrence, he or she should only correct contributing causes when the condition is high-risk/substandard. High-risk means that unless it's corrected, there is a high probability that the condition will result in a similar patient safety incident. Substandard means that the condition violates a core principle or value in the health care system.

### Questions to consider

*What if the root cause is outside of our control?*

Some analysts think that excluding causes outside of management's control to correct is unethical or maybe even immoral. But it is practical. RCA is not an activity performed for history. RCA is a learning activity used to make an informed decision to change the health care system and prevent future problems. Since we can only change what we can control, we should only consider possible root causes as those that we can control.

In most cases that involve a cause outside of management control, the analysts are examining the wrong half of the problem. Think of this in terms of a barrier analogy. A threat exists, so a barrier is provided to prevent the threat from causing harm. For example, on a pediatric unit where doses often vary with the patient's weight, physicians are at risk of making skill-based mistakes when performing dosing calculations in the medication ordering process. Skill-based slips and lapses are difficult to control. This is a threat to patient safety, so a hospital provides a barrier. Policy calls for a pharmacist to verify the calculation before the dose is dispensed and administered.

If the cause is outside of management control, consider it a threat and look for a barrier that is within management control. Case in point: A West Coast hospital lost telecommunications due to a heavy rainstorm. Asking why five times, the hospital arrived at rain as the root cause. But rain is normal in the system; rain is outside of management's control to correct or even influence. What about the leaking roof? That was the barrier within management's control, and the other half of the problem.

*Does the root cause always have to be cost-effective to correct?*

Yes. RCA is always intended to improve the system. This means that actions taken to fix the root cause conditions must have a positive net benefit to the system. The benefits in terms of direct cost savings of efficiency gained in the system and the indirect cost savings of improved patient safety, clinical quality, and patient satisfaction must outweigh the expense of the system changes and the cause analysis.

Estimate indirect costs using the following equation:

$$\text{Risk (\$/year)} = \text{Frequency of occurrence (events/year)} \times \text{Cost of losses (\$)}$$

If the system is improved, frequency of occurrence should decrease dramatically. Use quantitative methods for predicting human error probability to determine this decrease. You can estimate the cost of the following losses by accounting for the payouts associated with a patient safety event as a lower limit:

- Extended hospital stays
- Additional procedures and treatments
- Settlements
- Damage to hospital equipment
- Disgrace in the eyes of the community, etc.

*What if the state, regulator, accreditor, or insurer requires an action that is not cost-effective?*
Meeting commitments is part of the health care business. If you choose not to meet them, especially legal commitments, the only ethical course is to surrender the facility license and cease operations. With the extreme expense of closing in mind, those fixes look much more cost-effective.

This type of cost-effectiveness calculation can become truly problematic when we consider catastrophic failure modes that are very rare, especially in hospitals strapped for financial resources. Our country is facing this decision in deciding how much to invest in the health care system's capacity to respond to a bioterrorist attack.

*Why is it good for a root-cause condition to be substandard?*
A root cause condition doesn't need to be substandard, but one that is substandard provides tremendous reassurance to the root cause analyst that the condition is a root cause. Consider the case of a misguided hospital worker who took the last drag on a cigarette and threw the butt on to the floor. The butt rolled under the door of a housekeeping closet and set rolls of paper towels on fire. Smoke streamed down the corridor, a "code red" was sounded, fire doors closed, people scurried, and patients were moved to safety.

Let's use a fault tree to analyze this occurrence (see Figure 6.2). The fault tree is a cousin of the failure mode diagram. Failure mode diagrams have mutually exclusive possibilities; fault trees show synergistic effects using "and" and "or" logic gates. Recall from basic fire protection training that a fire requires three conditions in combination:

1. Fuel
2. Oxygen
3. Heat

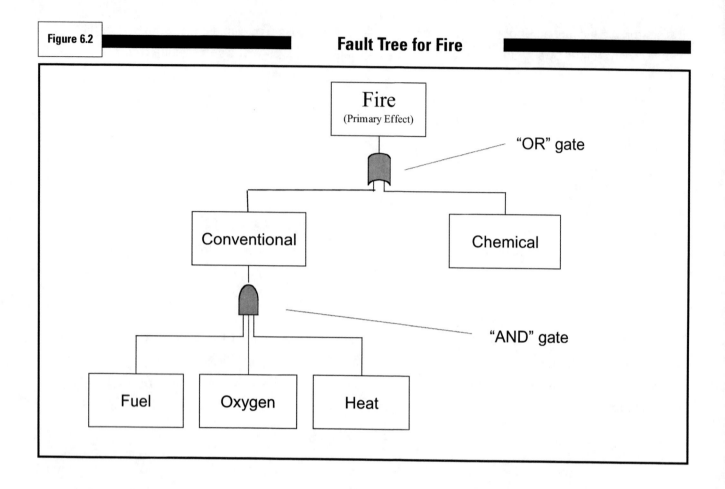

**Figure 6.2**  **Fault Tree for Fire**

Since fire requires all three elements, all three would be joined with an "and" gate. The three-factor approach made fire protection seem simple until we considered chemical fires, which don't require the combination of the three elements. This second class of fire would be shown with an "or" gate.

Use the fault tree just like a failure mode diagram by ruling out possibilities refuted by fact. The facts in the case rule out a chemical fire. Since conventional fire requires three elements in combination to occur and a root cause is something that if removed prevents recurrence, any one of the three could be a root cause. If we make oxygen the root cause, the corrective action for the hospital would be to have the entire facility inerted with nitrogen and all of the hospital employees (and patients) wear self-contained breathing apparati.

Test the root cause. Is there a proven cause-and-effect relationship between oxygen and fire? Yes. Is the corrective action within the control of management to implement? Yes. Is the corrective action cost-effective? No. Oxygen is not the root cause.

The good thing about RCA is that if you do it poorly you always get a second chance. Consider the paper towels. The purpose of the closet is to store the paper towels. Removing the towels may be in management's control and cost-effective, but the towels are not the substandard condition.

Only the cigarette butt is left. The cigarette butt is proven, within management control, cost-effective, and substandard. This cigarette butt is the path to a root cause. And while the substandard attribute of a root cause condition wasn't needed is this trivial case, in real cases we are not too sure.

Consider a case in which oversedation required the administration of a reversal agent. Patient alertness was not well-assessed during a moderate sedation procedure. There was a mismatch between the physician's knowledge and skill level and the detail in the moderate sedation flow sheet. Which is the root cause? The medical staff maintains that knowledge and skill levels are satisfactory; the flow sheet needs improvement. The hospital maintains the flow sheet is fine if the physicians knew what they were doing.

Use the same answer every time—the substandard condition. Take a look at the knowledge and skill level of the physicians. Examine the detail in the flow sheet. The one that is substandard is the path to root cause, and it is possible that both will be substandard.

If neither is substandard, treat the inappropriate action as an isolated error and focus the corrective actions on the individual. This statement has broad implications. Only substandard organizational, programmatic, human factor, work environment, and management failure modes can be root causes. If the standard is met, the system is not deficient and the cause of the occurrence is an isolated human error or equipment failure. Remember to always choose a good standard for comparison. Just because your hospital has the same performance as other hospitals it does not mean your performance acceptable. The best standard might be aviation for communication, as in crew-resource management, or high-tech manufacturing for automation, as in semiconductor manufacturing.

## Benchmarking

Benchmarking is the process of determining a standard. It can be performed by either process or result. Benchmarking by process is preferred because it is virtually impossible to compare results of measures due to the variability in data reporting, handling, and analysis. Benchmarking by process is determining a generally accepted method to accomplish a goal.

Benchmarking is a large topic to discuss well in short order. The following are quick tips about the process:

1. Search first for legal and regulatory requirements
2. Search next for consensus standards

3. Search last for published best practices and studies

4. If nothing is found, select a benchmarking group and collect data

## Why ask why?

Go back to the beginning of the RCA process. The root cause analyst first learns about the occurrence, followed by the primary effects, and then the failure modes. Could one of the failure modes also be a root cause? The only way to determine whether a failure mode is also a root cause is to test the failure mode. If the failure mode has all the attributes of a root cause, then it is a root cause.

If the failure mode does not have the attributes of a root cause, dig deeper into the failure scenario. Identify the next failure in the system. For inappropriate action, the system failure modes would be in the form of work environment, human factors, and organizational and programmatic (process). For work environment and human factors, the system failure modes are more likely organizational and programmatic and (occasionally) an isolated human error. For organizational and programmatic conditions, the system failure can be another organizational and programmatic failure mode but is most likely a management failure mode.

Keep using the process of identifying all possible failure modes and ruling them out with facts in the case to probe for conditions deeper and deeper in the failure scenario. Continue to do this until one of the failure modes has all three of the critical attributes of a root cause condition and perhaps the fourth as well.

Now that there is a failure mode that looks like a root cause, the question becomes, "Have I gone far enough or should I still go deeper?" The correct answer is a little more complicated than, "Ask why five times." The following are three different methods to determine whether the condition is the most basic one that, if corrected, prevents recurrence (i.e., the best failure mode that has the attributes of a root cause):

1. Compare the corrective action for each condition. If knowing the next, more basic condition does not change the corrective action, stop and designate the first condition as a root cause.

2. Determine the next, more basic condition. If it is more important than the previous, keep going. If the next condition is less important than the previous, stop and designate the condition at hand as a root cause.

3. Zero transportability method: If the condition (not the event) is isolated in the system, stop and designate the condition as a root cause.

## Handling multiple root causes

Using the failure mode diagrams, critical attributes for root causes, and three tests for comprehensiveness of the root causes makes the RCA sound very straightforward. However, complex systems such as health care are not always that straightforward. There are typically multiple inappropriate actions resulting in more than one root cause. A quick study of the last two years of PII's health care cases (183 cases) showed each occurrence had

- 8.8 inappropriate actions
- 2.2 root causes
- 1.6 contributing causes

Handle this complexity like a lawyer handles contributory negligence. Examine the contribution that each inappropriate action/equipment failure makes to the overall consequence. If an inappropriate action had minimal effect, treat the causes as either contributing factors or, in the case of very minimal contribution, a side issue in the cause analysis.

If an inappropriate action/equipment failure makes a substantial contribution to the consequence, treat the causes as root causes. But even here, look at the causes in terms of contribution to the inappropriate action or equipment failure. You need not correct all the causes. You must correct the set of causes that will prevent recurrence of the inappropriate action/equipment failure with a high degree of certainty. Those sets of causes are root causes and must have corrective actions. The other causes may be contributing causes and, if the causes are high-risk/substandard, also have a corrective action to prevent recurrence. The remaining causes may still be shown as a condition in the system that shaped behavior, but the causes should not have a corrective action.

## Summary

This chapter explained the importance of piecing together the story as part of your RCA. In the next chapter, we will take what we've learned so far and apply it to the next step: identifying the root solutions.

**Figure 6.3** ▬▬▬▬▬ **Three Rules for Root Cause Comprehensiveness** ▬▬▬

1. Monitor the corrective action for each condition. If knowing the next, more basic condition does not change the corrective action, stop and designate the condition as a root cause.

2. Question to the void: Determine the next, more basic condition. If the next condition is more important than the previous, keep going. If the next condition is less important than the previous, stop and designate the condition as a root cause.

3. Zero-transportability method: If the condition is isolated in the system, stop and designate the condition as a root cause.

**Figure 6.4** ▬▬▬▬▬ **Attributes of a Root Cause Condition** ▬▬▬

A root cause is a condition in the system that has the following critical attributes:

- The condition has a proven cause-and-effect relationship such that, if the condition is removed from the system, the occurrence is prevented and no harmful side-effects are created.

- The condition is within management's control to correct.

- The condition is cost-effective to correct.

* A root cause condition also has a fourth attribute that is good to have for confirmation: The condition is substandard.

| Figure 6.5 | ■■■■■■■■ "Attributes of a Contributing Cause" ■■■■■■■ |

A contributing cause is a condition in the system that has the following critical attributes:

- The condition has a proven cause-and-effect relationship such that the condition is known to increase the probability/severity of the occurrence. However, correcting the condition would not prevent recurrence.

- The condition is within management's control to correct.

- The condition is cost-effective to correct.

\* A root cause condition also has a fourth attribute that is good to have for confirmation: The condition is substandard.

# CHAPTER 7

## Develop Root Solutions

# CHAPTER 7

# Develop Root Solutions

## STEP 5

## What is a root solution?

In the previous chapter, we discussed identifying the root cause(s) that produce unwanted events. After you have identified the root cause(s) of your issue(s), you might assume that the hard work is done. However, we have found that even when organizations find the root cause(s) to their problems, they very often do not find the "root solution." The root solution to an event is that action or combination of actions that prevents the initial event its unwanted side-effects, and also prevents similar events in the future.

## Why is it so difficult to find root solutions?

There are two answers to this question that we will cover in this chapter:

1. Many organizations cannot distinguish individual performance issues v. system-driven issues. Therefore, the actions they take are too shallow to prevent recurrence of the event.

2. Many times correction efforts stop after the initial "broke-fix" actions are accomplished. These actions address symptoms and early compensatory measures to get things back to normal but, do not address the root cause of the problem.

## Individual v. system performance

Consider the model shown in Figure 7.1 on the following page. Most root cause analysis (RCA) investigations start with the identification of symptoms at the individual performance and equipment level of the

---

Performance Pyramid™. In other words, some of the first evidence that we collect comes from identifying problems in individual/equipment performance. These problems are often just symptoms of the actual problem. In fact, according to Dr. Edwards Deming, the highly respected quality guru mentioned earlier in the text, individual/equipment performance issues that drive quality problems are just symptoms more than 90% of the time. In our own research into significant events in many high-risk industries, we have found that individual and equipment performance issues are the root cause of events less than 15% of the time. The remaining 85% of the time the cause of an event lies in the organizational, programmatic, or management performance issues that influence or drive individual/equipment performance.

### Why does the system impact individual performance to such an extent?

There is no doubt that individuals commit mistakes due to fatigue, lack of attention, or intentional violation of rules. But for this type of thinking to explain the majority of errors that are committed, we would have to believe that if people are more careful, pay more attention, get more sleep, and follow the rules, then errors would cease to occur. However, this has been proven time and again not to be the case.

**Figure 7.1** ▬ **PII Performance Pyramid (A Comprehensive Event Reduction Model)** ▬

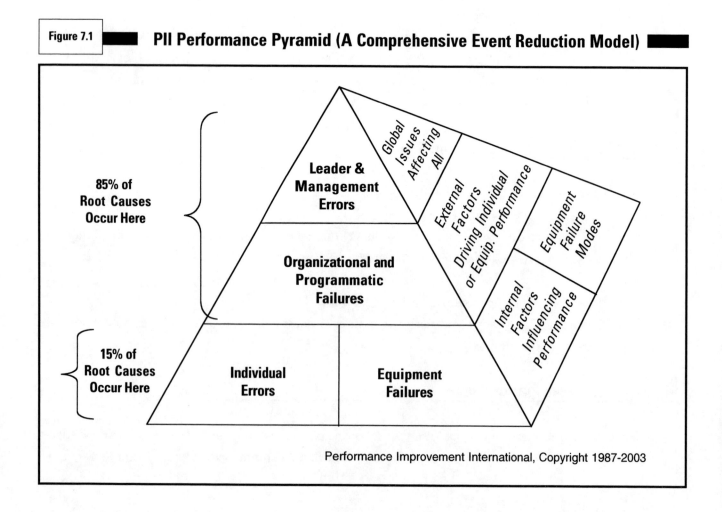

Performance Improvement International, Copyright 1987-2003

There are many simple cases that underscore how a system elicits a particular response from individuals performing within it. For example, North Americans who drive a car in England or Japan for the first time have a very difficult time overcoming the habits of a lifetime of driving on the right-hand side of the road.

They tend to glance to the right when looking for the image in the rear view mirror, expect to be passed on the left, and glance the wrong direction when looking for merging traffic. All of these behaviors are incorrect in those countries (in the "new" system); however, they are correct in their home country (the old system).

In the context of medical error, it is easy to find similar examples, such as: the labels on bottles may be very similar, and the connections on infusion pumps and equipment very confusing. This allows for staff to make potentially lethal interconnections. The layout of operating rooms may require wires, machinery, and supporting cables to run across the floor, causing tight conditions, trip hazards, and difficulty in communications during critical surgeries. Perhaps most notoriously, similarity in drug names and nomenclature provide ample opportunity for confusion and errors.

### How do we know what problem we are fixing?

You will correctly wonder whether you are fixing a system (shared) problem or individual performance issue. When studying inappropriate actions as a part of an investigation, you need to determine whether individual error is a contributing factor to the event. If it is, determine how often the error is seen. Then, compare that individual's performance to past situations, and against the performance of other individuals or groups of individuals performing same/similar functions within the same context. This will help determine the rate of occurrence and whether it is an internal (individual) or external (shared system-problem) factor that drove the error.

Most often it will not be possible to calculate the empirical rate of occurrence due to a lack of information regarding how often the actions performed were attempted. (To determine the empirical rate of occurrence would require the number of attempts performed v. the number performed in error.) This information is seldom available in statistical terms. However, it is possible to sample a workgroup by talking to others performing the same functions in similar environments within the same organization, to determine the frequency with which they also may have difficulty performing the task. It is also possible to benchmark with other organizations to determine the likelihood that performance problems are shared issues.

Once an effective problem-reporting and review system is in place, it is useful to look back at previous event history to determine the frequency with which similar problems have occurred.

If you lack information to support a diagnosis of the error as a shared issue, then you should apply corrective actions for individual error. These might include training, coaching or counseling, disciplinary action, mentoring, or observation by an experienced coworker. However, taking individual corrective actions should not limit you from looking at external factors that may have influenced individual performance, and implementing actions to fix significant external drivers.

When you find information during the investigation that points to an external factor or factors that drive numerous individual errors, the hospital will need to pursue system fixes rather than individual corrective actions. You can generally uncover this information through interviews with other individuals in the work group, a review of previous event history, review of organizational/programmatic factors that prove to be substandard by comparison to others, etc. This is not to say the individual has no culpability. Often, individual error triggers the scenario that leads to an event. But it does indicate that the root solution to the cause lies more with the system factors than individual performance issues.

## Pushing beyond 'broke-fix' actions: Remedial, compensatory, and preventive actions

The second reason that you may miss the mark in identification of root solutions has to do with how far you go in providing corrections. The following are three categories of actions associated with RCA:

- Remedial actions (immediate "broke-fix" actions)
- Compensatory actions (also referred to as interim corrections)
- Corrective actions to prevent recurrence (CATPR)

**Note:** These terms are also defined in **Chapter 11.**
Figure 7.2 represents the types of events that require each of these corrective actions.

The more significant the event, the more in-depth corrective actions are needed to preclude recurrence. And conversely, as shown in Figure 7.2, the less that is done to investigate the actual root cause of an event (as with lower-level issues), the less you should strive for actions to prevent recurrence (since a root cause has not been found).

### Remedial actions (immediate "broke-fix" actions)
Most organizations identify remedial actions rather easily, and are able to identify what remedial actions it must take to restore conditions to a safe and acceptable level.

---

| Figure 7.2 | **Corrective action applicability** |

| Problem Type | Remedial | Intermediate | To Prevent Recurrence |
|---|---|---|---|
| Significant (Root Cause) | Required | High Risk | Required |
| Less Significant (Apparent) | Required | High Risk | Avoid |
| Not Significant | Required | Avoid | Avoid |

In the case of administration of a penicillin injection to the wrong patient, the immediate action is to determine

1) will the patient who received the injection suffer a serious consequence (i.e., due to allergy)
2) provide the injection to the right patient

The problem you will find is that organizations stop with remedial corrective actions and do not press on to identify actions needed in the next two areas:

- Compensatory actions
- Corrective actions to prevent recurrence

### *Compensatory actions (also referred to as "interim" corrections)*
The next level of actions that results from an RCA involves compensatory actions taken to mitigate the consequences of inappropriate actions or defective systems before understanding the root cause. Often

---

these actions come from identifying the "extent of condition" or impact of the symptoms seen early in event recovery.

In the case of a patient who receives a mismatched blood type for transfusion due to a mislabeled batch of blood in the bank, compensatory measures may include sampling of blood supplies to determine the existence of other mislabeled batches.

It is worth noting that taking compensatory measures still does not address root cause, or provide a root solution. For instance, citing the example above, we still need to know why the blood products were mislabeled.

### Corrective actions to prevent recurrence (CATPR)

After the RCA team has determined the root cause(s) for the event, it needs to establish actions to prevent recurrence. These are the actions that will provide "root solutions" to the problems driving the event. For this reason, the team must aggressively evaluate the actions to determine whether they will be effective in eliminating the causes identified in the investigation. To make this determination, we have developed three tests you can apply to suggested actions.

In the previous chapter there were three main tests to determine whether the root cause selected was a good choice. These tests included the following:

1. The condition has a proven cause-and-effect relationship. In other words, if you remove the condition from the system, it will prevent the event of interest and harmful side effects.

2. The condition is within management's control to correct in a timely manner.

3. The condition is cost-effective to correct. In other words, it costs less to fix the problem than continue living with the deficiency.

You can apply these tests to the corrective actions selected to fix identified causes. For example:

- In evaluating question #1 above: If the action proposed to address a root cause condition does not preclude recurrence of that condition, it is not an effective action to prevent recurrence. Though performance may be improved, if there is no assurance that the event or similar occurrences cannot happen again, you must keep digging for a more fundamental, underlying action. Often when teams get to this point, they realize they may not have identified the root cause, since actions taken to address their causal statements will not preclude recurrence of the unwanted condition.

- In evaluating question #2 above: If actions suggested to correct conditions are effective in resolving the issue, but are not within the capability of assigned owners to implement, they are not likely to occur. What the assigned owner implements instead may ultimately be much less effective.

- In evaluating question #3 above: If actions suggested to correct conditions are effective in resolving the issue, but are not cost-effective (costs less to live with the problem or cannot be afforded at all), they are also not likely to occur. Root cause analysts must produce cost effective resolutions or the value in performing the investigation is lost to decision makers who must ultimately determine the course of action to take.

## Corrective action applicability

When determining the applicability of corrective actions, the type of error is the most important consideration. In previous chapters we discussed three types of human error: skill-based error, rule-based error, and knowledge-based error. The following are corrective actions proven through our research and that of other experts to be effective in addressing these types of errors.

### *Proven corrective actions for different human-error types (also refer to the discussion of error types in Chapter 11)*

1. Examples of proven corrective actions for skilled-based errors include

- Simplifying tasks, limiting memory requirements to five items at most, and standardizing signs, procedure format, forms, etc.
- Reducing distractions by workplace professionalism, uninterrupted periods involving critical work, and preparation of equipment, tools, and information before commencement of work
- Reducing unwanted time pressure through adequate staffing, good vertical communication, a high degree of trust among organizations, and good communications with supervisors
- Using awareness aids such as signs, pre-job meetings, and caution reminders periodically throughout critical procedures
- Maintaining an alert mental state through close supervision, good pre-job meetings, and failure symptom observation training
- Increasing experience for those performing critical tasks in high-stress, time-pressured environments
- Error-reduction training

2. Examples of proven corrective actions for rule-based errors include

- Work specialization

- Training in fundamentals by those who know the basis of the rules, not on-the-job training from those who do not
- Increased accountability
- Error-reduction training to improve the effectiveness of communications
- Use of QV&V to weed out bad information

3. Examples of proven corrective actions for knowledge based errors include

- Improved communication with more experienced performers
- Work specialization—focusing assignments based on previous knowledge and experience
- Improved problem solving skills
- Work process familiarization
- Knowledge-oriented training

## Summary

Why is it so much more difficult in cases of medical error to focus on system issues rather than individual performance in finding root solutions?

The answer lies in the discussion presented in the introduction: medical professionals work at the "Sharp End." The high level of dependency on individual knowledge and skill, combined with the sophistication of technology and medical devices make the administration of medicine more error-prone. And because of the very personal nature of how you administer care, the doctor, the nurse, and the technician all become central to the image we have of modern medicine.

The complexity of care, combined with the frequency of litigation, makes it much more consequential when errors are analyzed exclusively by those qualified in medicine, risk analysis or law, rather than those qualified to study error and its causes.

## The next step

You are not finished just because you have identified corrective actions. One of the easiest ways to fail in performing RCA is to quit too soon. You still must make sure each corrective action recommended lands in the capable hands of an individual or group manager for implementation.

Chapter 8 describes how you can be sure to fix problems the first time, making certain that they don't happen again. You might ask, "How important is this?" Answer: The results of one case study from another high-risk/high-complexity industry showed of the 28 commercial nuclear plants that were shut down by the regulator for problems related to performance, 22 of the shutdowns were caused by ineffective review, investigation, and corrective actions from previous significant events and incidents.

The path you are on has been traveled by other industries before you. Just as we have seen in those other industries, your ability to "hold the gains" achieved from your RCA efforts will ultimately determine who wins and who fails.

# CHAPTER 8

## Monitor for Effectiveness—
## The Last Step

# CHAPTER 8

# Monitor for Effectiveness— The Last Step

**STEP 6**

Monitoring the effectiveness of the corrective actions is the last step in this six-step process. It is intended to prevent recurrence of the condition that caused the event. Root cause analysis (RCA) teams often overlook this step because they have long since identified the root causes. However, ensuring that the health care system is changed for the better by these corrective actions is the most critical step in the process.

A study by PII found that even organizations that perform good RCAs require between four and eight attempts (RCAs with that cause present) to correctly diagnose the cause and extent of condition for global system problems. Most organizations churn the training programs and the policies and procedures without ever addressing the system problems. Poor RCA organizations require more than 20 related events, and some organizations never successfully correct global system problems.

## It is important to monitor for effectiveness

Monitoring for effectiveness is critical because, sadly, most corrective actions do not work well the first time. Be prepared to adjust the corrective actions during implementation, and be prepared to institute an alternate corrective action plan in cases where the primary plan fails.

## The corrective action tracking system

Each RCA should have a plan to monitor effectiveness of the corrective actions in the RCA report. The simplest method, although not the most effective, is a corrective action tracking system. Tracking corrective actions to completion ensures that the corrective actions are in fact completed on time. Before you close the case, ensure that the hospital completed the corrective action as intended.

Base the due date of a specific corrective action on the urgency to patient safety and the importance of the problem. However, the following two measures are useful for judging overall corrective action timeliness:

1. Average age of all corrective actions is less than 180 days.
   Note: In this instance, average age means the average time between when the corrective action is created and when the corrective action is completed.

2. 90% of all corrective actions are completed on or before the due date.

## Use two tracking measures to ensure accurate monitoring results

Tracking corrective actions and monitoring timeliness of the corrective action implementation are critical success factors of effective RCA programs. (Please see **Chapter 9** for more details about this.) Using two measures prevents staff from gaming the system. If you used only the on-time measure, the staff could extend the due dates so that all actions are completed on time. If you use only the average age measure, overdue actions would hide among the few, simple actions that were completed very quickly. Using two measures makes the measurement system very difficult to trick.

## Create a follow-up action

In order to ensure the results that the RCA team intended, create a follow-up action that assesses the behavior change effected by the corrective actions. The following are two basic methods to assess:

1. Perform a monitoring self-assessment of the system
2. Create a measure of the system performance

See Figure 8.1 for an example of both methods. This figure also includes the recommended number of root cause cases for which you should use each method. A monitoring self-assessment is less effective in measuring results, but much more efficient for the organization to perform.

**Tip:** Use the monitoring self-assessment in 80% of the cases. The system measure is very effective in gauging results, but requires more people and time. Use the system measure in the other 20% of cases, especially the more important cases.

Perform the monitoring self-assessment by creating a follow-up action to be performed at a suitable date after corrective action implementation. For example, in a case where corrective action required that the team created and communicated behavior-based expectations for patient identification, members scheduled

Figure 8.1 **Two Methods for Monitoring Corrective Action Effectiveness**

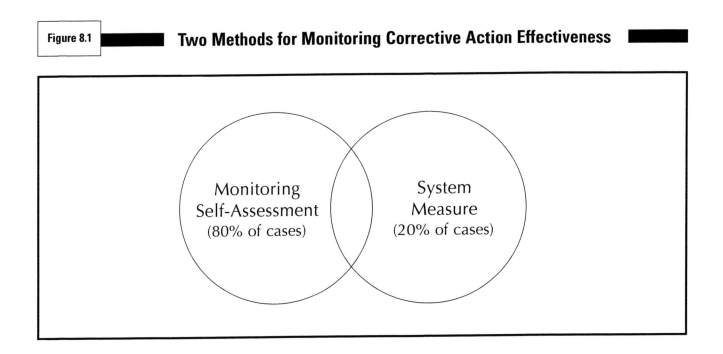

Monitoring
Self-Assessment
(80% of cases)

System
Measure
(20% of cases)

the follow-up for six months after they completed the communication plan. One or two of the original root cause analysts would then collect objective evidence to judge the effectiveness of the action.

## Make sure the assessment monitors behavior

Best results are obtained when the monitoring self-assessment observes the behavior changes associated with the corrective action. Behaviors are easier to observe than results, and behaviors are also more indicative of performance than interview statements. Create a small set of objective assessment criteria, choose a sample of the professional groups, units, etc., for the assessment, and collect the data using standard observation techniques. As a simplifying hint, use the same standard for accepting the change that you used to establish the condition as a substandard during the RCA.

## Focus the measures on behavior

Focus the measures on behavior, just as you focused the monitoring self-assessments on behavior. Behavior tends to be a real-time measure of performance. The performance culture that drives behavior tends to be a leading measure of performance; sentinel event rate tends to be a very lagging measure of performance. Figure 8.2 shows a typical event pyramid. For each actual event where there is loss of life/serious loss of property, there tends to be 12,000 unsafe behaviors on average. It would be better to detect an adverse trend by measuring unsafe behavior rather than the loss of life. This focuses perform-ance improvement on prevention, rather than addressing an event, especially a serious one that involves loss of life. Moreover, despite the fact that it might be easier to measure loss of life, this should be such an infrequent occurrence that it cannot be a sensitive measure of whether or not your organization is improving.

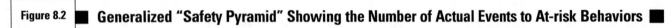

**Figure 8.2** ■ **Generalized "Safety Pyramid" Showing the Number of Actual Events to At-risk Behaviors** ■

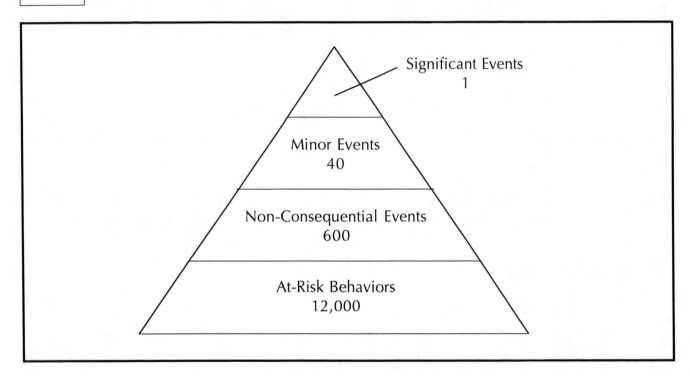

## Case study: Near miss event

*Consider a case from a large, Midwestern surgical center as an example. This case was a near miss-event in wrong-patient surgery.*

*Dr. Burton (not the surgeon's real name) was performing a series of four procedures at one hospital before leaving for rounds at a nearby hospital. Upon finishing the second, the circulating nurse called for Dr. Burton's next case. The surgical technician checked the board, identified the patient, and delivered the next patient. Dr. Burton was strong in patient identification; she immediately recognized that the patient was the fourth case (biopsy) instead of the third case (mastectomy). The technician had just brought in Dr. Burton's next case on the board. He had bypassed two process controls that would have correctly identified the third case.*

### RCA findings in the case study

*The RCA found several similar inappropriate actions and eventually focused on system problems leading to poor knowledge of job standards and noncompliance. Six months after the hospital completed the corrective actions, two nurses from the quality department performed a series of observations in the surgical center to verify that the actions were effective in changing the behaviors. The nurses observed for the following:*

1. *Nurses calling for patients by name, surgeon, and procedure*
2. *Technicians using a repeat-back to confirm information transmission*
3. *Technicians verifying the case on the surgical schedule*
4. *Technicians locating the correct chart based on patient name, surgeon, and procedure*
5. *Technicians performing patient identification using the chart as the controlling document and the name and date of birth on the identification bracelet*
6. *Nurses verifying the surgical site marking is correct per the chart and consent*

*Since each action is routine and performed in a familiar environment, a slip-and-lapse error probability was used as a standard. The standard selected was three errors per every 1,000 actions or 0.3%. This effectively meant zero inappropriate actions in the sample, which was the result of the monitoring self-assessment. The RCA case was deemed a success, and the hospital closed the case.*

## When to use the system measure

Use the system measure in the other 20% of cases, especially the more important cases that tend to be global systems problems. For these cases, develop a performance measure that indicates that success of the corrective actions. Have a follow-up action in the RCA that provides for the measure, management control loop surrounding the measure, and a goal for the measure. For global systems, a reasonable goal is an 80% reduction in error rate over the implementation period of the action, which for large hospitals may be as long as two years.

### Case study: Three event types

*Consider a case from a large, Midwestern hospital as an example. In this case the root causes were common causes of several event types: medication administration, coordinating care, monitoring patient condition, etc. One of the more significant causes was communication, which the RCA team learned was due to poor communication channels (a process problem) and poor professional standards for repeat-back, clarifying questions, and critical thinking (organizational problems). The corrective action plan included several improvement initiatives and a measure (the number of adverse events in which communication was a contributing factor or cause) with a goal of 80% reduction in two years. The patient safety committee, which provided oversight to the corrective action plan, developed a management control loop.*

#### Effectiveness of the corrective action plan in the case study

*In the first three months of the corrective action plan, the reduction in adverse events was on schedule so the plan continued as written. In the second quarter of the plan, the improving trend reversed. The team added corrective actions to the plan and accelerated some future actions (technology for instant messaging). The third quarter result showed that the results were again on track per the goal. This case is still ongoing with a promising outcome. However, the positive outcome would have not been possible without the effectiveness measure, the control loop, and the additional corrective actions.*

## Holding the gains

The cartoon character Pogo is widely credited with the observation, "We have met the enemy and he is us." This statement is very much true with regard to the challenges of implementing good corrective actions. PII's experience in health care has found that four issues influence hospital administration to defer, deflate, and delete corrective actions to improve their own systems. The following are the four leading causes of corrective action death in health care:

1. Hidden noncommitment
2. Soft cost-benefit analysis
3. Medical staff resistance
4. Poor implementation accountability

Hidden noncommitment is evident when administration agrees to the corrective action plan to complete the cause analysis and then spends the next six-months trying to back-out of the plan. This effect is best dealt with as an RCA process problem. Managers in the hospital should take responsibility for RCA of significant events. Patient safety and quality organizations do not perform RCA on us; we (management) do it for ourselves through RCA teams.

Ideas to consider include the following:

- Keep managers engaged in corrective action plan development

- Use the sponsor of the root cause team to negotiate the corrective actions with other leaders who will implement the corrective actions

- Literally sign up each manager accountable for implementation before finishing the RCA report.

- Ensure that each corrective action has the attributes of a root solution and is
    - proven to prevent recurrence without harmful side effects
    - within management control to implement
    - cost effective

If the root solution has all three attributes, what manager would block the implementation of the corrective action?

## Factors in the downfall of the correction plan

Soft cost-benefit analysis is the leading killer of marginal corrective action plans. Administrators want to do the right thing, but their thinking can only be stretched so far without the support of the health care economic model. Ideally, a root solution is always cost-effective. This means that the direct costs of implementation are less than the cost savings of the solution. Cost savings are in the form of direct savings (from efficiency gains) and indirect savings (reducing extended hospital stays, unrecoverable treatment fees, settlement costs, etc.)

Dr. Philip Crosby, another father of the quality movement, said quality is free. What he meant was that quality (and patient safety) is an investment that pays. The best way to show the payoff is to provide an economic analysis of the corrective action plan. Estimate the costs of implementation and compare to the estimated costs of failure. Include all of the four D's in the cost of failure: death, destruction, dose (chemical and radiological exposure), and disgrace (in the eyes of the community and regulators). The two largest assumptions will be the probability of future failures and the expected reduction in this failure rate. Here, PII suggests using probabilistic risk assessment (PRA) and quantitative methods to predict human error rate.

Remember, the objective in providing the cost-benefit analysis is not always to demonstrate a payback greater than the hurdle rate for the hospital. Sometimes the objective of the analysis is to make the corrective action plan look good enough to pass as the "right thing to do."

### The effect of poor accountability on the correction plan

Poor accountability for implementation kills good corrective actions—only this death is one of neglect. While accountability is an organizational culture trait (meaning responsibility to meet expectations or standards), this accountability problem is primarily a process problem. Good accountability systems invariably lead to good accountability.

Assign each corrective action to an implementation manager by name. Assign all corrective actions with a due date. Monitor both the average age of the corrective actions and the timeliness of completion relative to the assigned dates. Have an overdue list that is monitored by the patient safety officer or the patient safety committee. Due date extensions are acceptable, but each extension requires a progressively higher approval authority. The quality director authorizes the first extension, for example. The second would be approved by a vice president, and the third extension requires the CEO. Not many managers look forward to the third extension.

There should be a method to ensure that corrective action owners are accountable without the omnipresent threat of the overdue list. But not many organizations use that method. One West Coast facility had an innovative approach to implementing accountability—there was no overdue list or timeliness measure. Every Friday at 5 p.m., all managers with overdue corrective actions lined up outside of administration offices. The CEO patiently worked with each manager to find solutions to overcome the implementation challenge.

The managers quickly came to understand that maybe a good manager doesn't need this kind of help from the CEO on Friday afternoon. The CEO was always supportive and encouraging but the point was clear. Good safety culture means getting your corrective actions done on time every time.

## Convincing the medical staff: Getting them on board with the correction plan

The medical staff will make or break any substantive change to patient care. Rely on tactful diplomacy. Identify interested physicians early in the RCA process. Educate them on the facts in the case and solicit their input into possible solutions. Continue this communication process throughout the analysis. Put special emphasis on the science behind the system failure and the proven solutions to prevent recurrence. Educated people will draw the same conclusion when presented with the same facts.

Dr. Frank Carlton, MD the medical director of clinical quality improvement and the patient safety officer at Memorial Health University Medical Center in Savannah, GA, expressed this point well. "Physicians are trained as scientists; they respond well to credible data presented in support of improved patient care." They tend not to respond to emotional appeals for the greater good of health care, says Carlton. "Be polite, work through the opinion leaders, and ask before mandating action and most physicians will do the right thing."

Seek approval of any change that affects the medical staff through the proper committees and departments. There is no one decision-maker, identify the physicians (opinion leaders) whose support is critical for acceptance of the proposed change and gain their approval.

## What motivates the physicians

Physicians have a strong professional culture. They care deeply about their patients and the quality of care that their patients receive. They are motivated by knowledge and excellence for themselves, their profession, and their hospital. Physicians are also, by in large businesspeople who must make their own business models work. They measure the success of their day in 30-second increments of time that other people waste for them. Forms, protocols, and requests appear at an alarming rate. Insurance premiums are skyrocketing and the liability crisis mounts. They desperately want the hospital to change (for the better) but cannot bear the thought of one more change at the hospital.

There is a success path. Emphasize the positives: patient care, excellence, and success. Avoid, or at least neutralize the hot buttons: time, burden, and change. These edges will give the best probability of gaining physician approval of a good root solution. Always make your solution a good root solution. There is no best probability of gaining approval for a poor root solution.

# CHAPTER 9

# How to Establish
# a High-Performing
# Cause-Analysis Program

# CHAPTER 9

## How to Establish a High-Performing Cause-Analysis Program

### The 25 elements of a high-performing cause-analysis program

Your hospital's quality improvement program cannot be successful without an effective cause analysis program.

An effective cause-analysis program is composed of the following five phases:

- **Initiation**—identifying the problem, notifying appropriate hospital leaders about the issue, preserving physical evidence, and performing any necessary remedial corrective actions.

- **Screening**—determining the severity of the event and how much analysis is required.

- **Analysis**—assigning the investigation to a responsible individual, establishing the root cause analysis (RCA) team, and conducting the RCA

- **Implementation**—presenting the results of the investigation to appropriate management personnel for approval and putting the agreed-upon corrective actions into place within the specified time frame.

- **Monitoring**—verifying that the hospital fixed the problem and that the corrective actions also help prevent similar events due to the same causes.

We describe each of these five phases by a collection of "success factors," which guide us in the development of an effective cause analysis program. You can also use them to perform an assessment of an existing program to identify opportunities for improvement. Five success factors describe each phase of the process for a total of 25 factors. These factors are visually provided in Figure 9.1 and are briefly described on the next page.

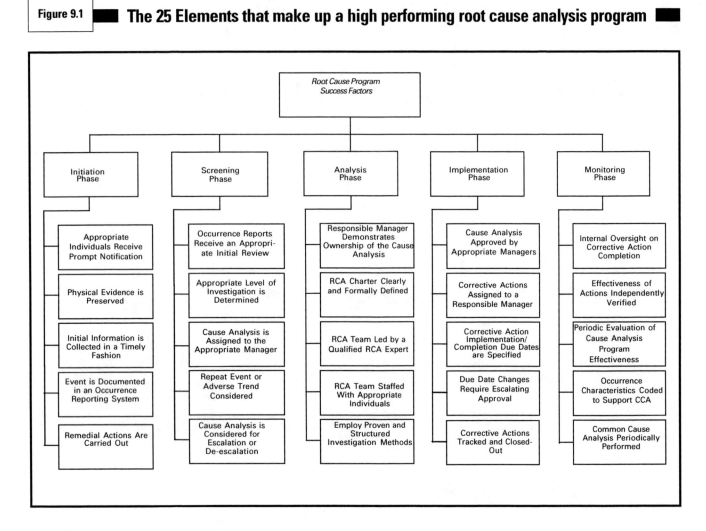

## Initiation phase

### 1. Appropriate individuals receive prompt notification of an event

An organization cannot solve its problems until it knows about them. When an event occurs, individuals must promptly report it to appropriate leaders, such as the department manager or the attending physician. Supervisors and managers must take a nonpunitive approach to those involved in the event and those who reported the occurrence. If managers place inappropriate blame on individuals, those who witness an event won't report problems.

### 2. Physical evidence is preserved

For significant near-miss events or sentinel events that will require a formal RCA, it is important to preserve any relevant physical evidence. Organizations must quarantine any equipment that is directly involved or may be related to the cause(s) of the event. If the equipment is defective and taken out of service, it will not cause another similar problem. The quarantined equipment will be available to those conducting the RCA. If appropriate, document the "as-found" state of the equipment, such as machine settings. Sometimes it is useful to photograph or videotape a scene to preserve information for further study.

### 3. Initial information is collected in a timely fashion

Gather known information pertinent to the event, such as what happened, who was involved, and the sequence of events. Briefly describe what was seen, heard, or felt. Identify any relevant environmental conditions or external factors that might have contributed to the event. If possible, note the mental states of those involved. Were they under stress, fatigued, confused, or overconfident?

### 4. Event is documented in an occurrence-reporting system

Organizations should have a preestablished method (such as an occurrence-reporting system) for individuals to use to report incidents. Individuals should report events as soon as possible and practical after the discovery of the problem. In all cases, the person who discovers the problem should file a report before the end of his or her shift. The report should include the event date/time, location, consequences, a brief description of what happened, who was involved, why the person submitting the report thinks the event happened, and what actions (remedial measures) were taken after the incident.

### 5. Remedial actions are carried out

Immediate evaluation of the situation includes the extent of the condition and identification of necessary remedial actions. If appropriate, the organization should take interim actions to minimize the short-term risk of a similar event.

### *Screening phase*

### 6. Occurrence reports receive an initial review by appropriate individuals

A small group of individuals or a committee should conduct a timely review of all events disclosed during the occurrence reporting process. The initial review should determine risk significance and appropriate organizational response.

### 7. Appropriate level of investigation is determined

Organizations should conduct a formal RCA for sentinel events, other significant incidents, and events management considers worthy of spending scarce RCA money and resources. Less consequential events should receive an apparent-cause analysis. Either way, organizations must collectively analyze all events using a common cause analysis or an analogous technique on a periodic basis to identify adverse trends.

### 8. Cause analysis is assigned to the appropriate manager

Cause analysis is the responsibility of line management. It must not be "owned" by a staff support department such as quality improvement or risk management. Although those areas should provide root cause expertise to individual departments, the responsibility to deliver a quality cause analysis must remain with the culpable department. Therefore, it is critical that the organization assign responsibility for the cause analysis to a responsible manager, such as the manager of the department where the problem occurred. Assignment should normally occur within 24 hours of discovery of the problem.

### 9. Repeat event or adverse trend considered

When an individual reports an occurrence, the person assigned to analyze the event should also consider past incidents of a similar type. If similar events occurred in the past, the organization may want to undergo a root cause evaluation for a relatively minor incident.

### 10. Cause analysis is considered for escalation or de-escalation

As facts become available during an apparent-cause analysis, it may be necessary to escalate the analysis to a formal RCA. Similarly, an organization may want to de-escalate an RCA to an apparent-cause analysis if facts uncovered early in the investigation indicate this is appropriate.

### *Analysis phase*

### 11. Responsible manager demonstrates ownership of the RCA

The individual assigned ownership of the RCA (typically not the investigation team leader) must support the investigation with appropriate resources and management attention. This individual is ultimately responsible to the organization for the quality of the cause analysis and the appropriateness of the corrective actions or other improvement recommendations.

### 12. RCA charter is clearly and formally defined

When an RCA is initiated, the process should require the development of an investigation "charter." This document should clearly identify the analysis scope, schedule, and deliverables. In addition, the charter should call for managers to formally assign an investigation team leader and team members to conduct the investigation.

### 13. RCA team is led by a qualified RCA expert

RCA requires specific skills and experience. Individuals who lead root cause investigations should have the appropriate mix of personal attributes, formal training in basic and advanced RCA techniques, and developed abilities through on-the-job training. Therefore, qualified and experienced individuals should lead root cause investigations.

### 14. RCA team staffed with appropriate individuals

The team performing an RCA should consist of appropriate subject-matter experts and management personnel. Smaller investigation teams are usually a better choice. The majority of members will function as "part-time" participants when the team performs investigation activities. This will serve to minimize impact on participating individuals' time and will also ensure appropriate representation on the cause-analysis team.

### 15. Employ proven and structured investigation methods

The team should use objective, proven, and evidence-based investigation methods during the cause analysis. Subjective techniques, such as brainstorming, can provide general focus and issue development, but are not a reliable or efficient means of determining root solutions.

### *Implementation phase*

### 16. Cause analysis is approved by appropriate manager(s)

Management should approve and accept the final cause-analysis report and corrective action plan. These managers should know critical characteristics of a high-quality RCA. In addition, they should understand appropriate and effective corrective actions for the identified root cause(s).

### 17. Corrective actions are assigned to a responsible manager for implementation

The organization must assign all corrective actions (remedial, interim, and corrective actions to prevent recurrence) to a specific manager or individual to carry out.

### 18. Corrective action implementation/completion due dates are specified

The report must specify a due date or completion date for all corrective actions. Track the actions and report progress to appropriate managers.

### 19. Corrective-action due-date extensions require escalating approval

The organization should establish a predefined process for granting due-date extensions to committed corrective action completion dates. Additional extensions require approval at higher levels in the organization.

### 20. Corrective actions tracked and closed-out

Perform the tracking and verification of completed corrective actions as a central function. Submit periodic reports of corrective action status to appropriate management personnel. Individuals responsible for following through on the actions should provide documents that certify they completed the corrective measures. Real-time status of commitments should be available to those responsible for completion of corrective actions.

### *Monitoring phase*

### 21. Internal oversight on corrective action completion

The organization should conduct periodic, internal audits to verify that individuals completed mission-critical corrective actions. A sampling audit should be sufficient unless the auditor identifies significant deficiencies, in which case the organization may want to conduct 100% verification.

### 22. Effectiveness of corrective actions is independently verified

RCAs should provide a method to verify that specified corrective actions did in fact prevent recurrence of the incident. Monitoring self-assessments are effective for individual corrective actions. Common cause analysis is a useful technique to verify actions in aggregate.

### 23. Periodic evaluation of cause analysis program effectiveness

The organization should conduct a periodic self-assessment on the cause-analysis program for effectiveness. The 25 attributes presented in this section provide an initial guide for this assessment. You could rate each attribute as "green" or strength, "yellow" or an opportunity for improvement, or "red," a significant area of concern.

### 24. Occurrence characteristics and inappropriate actions categorized to support common cause analysis

The organization should characterize each occurrence report and analysis (root cause and apparent cause) in specific dimensions to facilitate the performance of a periodic common-cause analysis. These dimensions include: organization or professional group, work process, key activity, human error type, human error failure mode, organizational/programmatic failure mode, high-risk situation, and high-risk behavior. The organization should assign one or two trained evaluators to characterize the information to ensure consistency and accuracy.

### 25. Common cause analysis is periodically performed

At least once a year, the organization should conduct a common cause analysis on all events reported through the occurrence reporting system that identify human performance issues. The organization should perform formal RCA on significant issues identified during the common-cause analysis.

## Evaluating the effectiveness of your cause-analysis program

Certain parameters will indicate the effectiveness of your cause-analysis program. A top-performing organization routinely monitors performance indicators to ensure the cause-analysis program is working well. Typical indicators include the following:

### • Significant event rate trend

One true indicator of a healthy quality-improvement and cause-analysis program is the rate of significant events, such as sentinel events or legal claims, over time. Continuous improvement of this trend indicates a healthy cause-analysis program.

### • Event or occurrence reporting threshold

Establish clear expectations for reporting events in the organization. Individuals should report any condition adverse to quality care so that the organization can take appropriate remedial actions and conduct an appropriate cause analysis (root or apparent cause). Industries that conduct high-risk activities and have a healthy cause-analysis program receive reports of between seven and 20 minor (low consequence or no consequence) events for each significant occurrence that needs an RCA. Because the causes of minor events and significant events are statistically similar, this ratio ensures that organizations have an adequate numbers of events to perform common-cause analysis.

### • RCA threshold

Management should establish and define in hospital policies an appropriate threshold for formal RCA based on safety/economic significance of the event. This threshold should result in the following outcomes:

- Hospital personnel or physicians should report all significant occurrences, such as sentinel events, into the occurrence-reporting system. Hospital management should not learn of these events from an outside entity, such as a patient, a plaintiff's attorney, or others.

- The organization should perform an adequate number of RCAs. It's important to use RCA as an effective improvement tool—not just one used to meet regulatory requirements. Therefore, an organization with a healthy self-improvement culture performs more optional root cause investigations than those required by regulation or actual patient harm.

For example, if a hospital has a healthy self-improvement culture, 60% to 90% of the RCA it performs are optional. In other words, the hospital elects to conduct the optional RCAs and is not required to do so by regulators or outside agencies such as the Joint Commission on Accreditation of Healthcare Organizations (JCAHO). Hospitals that approach the threshold of "90% optional" RCA do so because of their low rate of required RCA. They commit a certain amount of organizational resources to support RCA. As the organizations' significant event rates requiring RCA improves they perform a greater percentage of "optional" RCAs.

### • Apparent-cause analysis quality

An apparent-cause analysis is a limited investigation of an event that is often performed instead of an RCA for less significant incidents. An apparent-cause analysis should require less than an hour to complete as opposed to a formal RCA, which might require weeks. Apparent-cause analysis is a process to identify remedial corrective actions and information necessary to support future common-cause analyses. We strongly discourage organizations to take corrective action(s) to prevent recurrence if an organization only performs an apparent-cause analysis because it doesn't know the true root causes. The following attributes are present in high-quality apparent-cause analyses

- Briefly describes the event that addresses all conditions that are adverse to quality and includes what did happen (and what should have happened if not apparent), who was involved, and when/where the problem occurred

- Considers actual and potential safety consequences of the specific event and the extent of condition beyond the incident

- Includes remedial corrective actions for all identified conditions adverse to quality

- Identifies obvious inappropriate actions and provides a brief description as to why the error occurred based on immediately available facts, not based on a formal RCA

- Avoids taking or judiciously applying corrective actions to prevent recurrence if the organization didn't perform a formal RCA

- Identifies corrective action implementation due dates (and the person or group responsible for carrying them out) for any measure not immediately taken in response to the event

## • RCA quality

A high-quality RCA report embodies the following characteristics:

- Includes all relevant facts and supports the conclusions of the report

- Develops all the critical facts through the Qualification, Validation, and Verification (QV&V) process

- Determines (with supporting facts) that an isolated human error, a localized organization/program-matic issue, or a management issue caused the event

- Considers all inappropriate actions, failed barriers, and failure modes when determining the root cause(s)

- Only identifies barriers that have a high degree of reliability in preventing the event as an area of root cause

- Doesn't provide narrow or inappropriately focused corrective actions

- Proves that the identified organizational/programmatic causes were substandard when compared to other similar organizations or processes

- Doesn't rely solely on interviewee statements to identify significant organizational or programmatic issues, but demonstrates substandard performance through additional means, such as documents or benchmarking

- Considers similar events that occurred previously to check for cause analysis failures and repeat events

- Assesses the ineffectiveness of previous corrective actions implemented for similar events to ensure that the organization doesn't take the same inappropriate corrective actions

### • Self-identification performance ratio

It is important for each department in a hospital or organization to "own" its problems, or be self-critical. One parameter that indicates this level of commitment is called the self-identification performance ratio (SIPR). In this context, the term "self" indicates the organization itself, not an individual person. The following equation mathematically expresses SIPR:

$$SIPR = \frac{\text{\# of occurrence reports generated by a department and assigned to that department as culpable}}{\text{\# of occurrence reports generated by all departments and assigned to that department as culpable}}$$

As this ratio approaches zero, it indicates that an organization is not self-identifying problems. As the ratio moves toward one, it indicates that an organization is self-identifying more problems. The desired ratio is > 0.5 and improving over the previous period.

### Investigation initiation timeliness

The sooner an organization initiates the cause analysis, the better. Time is of the essence. For this reason, most organizations strive to start the formal cause investigation within 24 hours of event or problem discovery. However, as mentioned earlier in this chapter, organizations should begin to immediately collect initial information upon discovering the problem.

### Investigation completion timeliness

The investigation or RCA should take the time required: no more, no less. Most organizations strive to complete the RCA in a time frame consistent with regulations and prudent business practices. A typical goal is to complete the cause analysis through management approval of the report and corrective action plan within 30 to 45 days. An apparent cause investigation is fairly straightforward and based on readily available information so a typical goal is seven days. However, some organizations allow up to 45 days for the completion of an apparent-cause analysis.

### Corrective action implementation timeliness

To avoid future events due to the same cause, it's important that organizations put approved corrective actions in place in a timely manner. Therefore, an organization must be judicious in committing to these actions, but then must be aggressive in completing the corrective measures. A typical goal in other industries with a healthy self-improvement culture is to complete corrective actions within 90–180 days depending on their scope and complexity. In addition, a goal of 90% of all corrective actions completed on or before the original due date should be established.

## Summary

This chapter explained the 25 elements that make up a high-performing cause analysis program (see Figure 9.1). In the next chapter, we will discuss the importance of including common cause analyses in your program.

# CHAPTER 10

# Breakthrough to
# Common-Cause Analysis

# CHAPTER 10

---

# Breakthrough to Common-Cause Analysis

To manage and improve performance in a complex system such as health care, organizations need more information to describe the system problems than a single event can provide. Each event, significant or not, describes a symptom of a latent weakness in the system. much like a piece of a jigsaw puzzle describes the picture on the puzzle. The more pieces to the puzzle that you have, the more effective you will be in improving the system.

## Common-cause analysis

Common cause analysis is more powerful than traditional single-event root cause analysis (RCA) because it provides more information that describes problems in the system. A study of the effectiveness of common-cause analysis performed by PII found that a common-cause analysis program has the same effectiveness in reducing event rates (and safety, quality, and production losses) as the entire RCA program with only 10% of the resource allocation.

The phrase "common cause" has two different meanings, and both are important in performing RCA in health care. Common cause can refer to a local or global system problem that is the reason for multiple events. The multiple occurrences typically have similar consequences, such as a cluster of medication ordering errors or an adverse trend in risk assessment for patient falls. In this usage "common cause" translates as a shared root cause(s) (i.e., the events have common root causes).

Events, occurrences, and errors don't need similar consequences to have common causes. They typically do because we often choose a particular set of occurrences for analysis *because* they each had that particular consequence. We choose to examine medication ordering errors together; or we choose to examine adverse trends in risk assessment for patient falls. We could also decide to examine a set of apparently

---

unrelated occurrences for common cause. This would be more like a hospitalwide common-cause analysis in which all significant events (sentinel events and other near-miss events deemed worthy of RCA) are simultaneously analyzed.

You could also apply this approach at the organizational or process level. For example, an organization could conduct a common-cause analysis of all the occurrences that took place during the start-up of a new cardiac unit at a large medical center or a common-cause analysis of all patient falls with injury in nursing units.

### Common-cause variation

The second use of the phrase "common cause" is derived from the theory of variation. Complex systems have a great deal of inherent variation, and health care is no exception. Consider the following: Two patients are admitted to a hospital on the same day with the same diagnosis. Both receive the same treatment from the same doctors, nurses, and technicians. One patient does well on that course of treatment and is discharged after four days and the other lingers with complications: He is admitted to a higher-acuity unit for a few days, transferred to a step-down unit, and remains at the hospital after 10 days. This variability would drive Six Sigma quality organizations insane, but it is par for the course in health care.

In the theory of variation, outcomes fluctuate for better and worse with occasional sharp spikes in bad outcomes. The sharp spikes represent specific or assignable causes. As a result, organizations respond and perform traditional RCA, carry out recommendations, and the system returns to normal. But what is normal? No one ever said that the normal number of patient falls per adjusted patient days is acceptable. In fact, organizations should do everything they can to reduce the number of falls while maintaining a healthy balance among overall patient safety, clinical quality, and patient satisfaction, and allocation of health care resources.

The inherent variation in the system—the normal number of problems—is representative of common causes. (See Figure 10.1 for a visual depiction of specific and common causes.)

| Figure 10.1 | **Graphical Representations of Specific and Common Causes Resulting in Loss Events** |

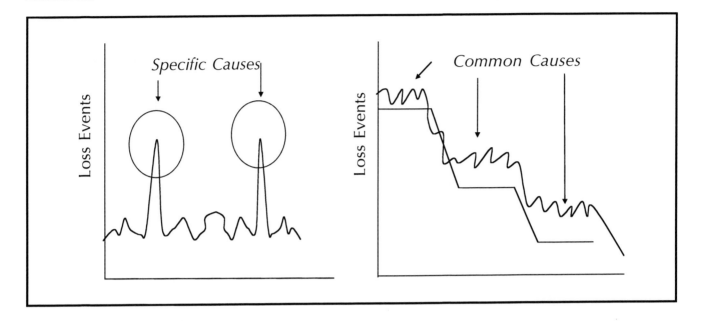

Since there is no acceptable number for problems, how do you diagnose and correct a common cause? Traditional cause analysis approaches are fairly explicit for specific causes, but much less so for common causes. Organizations remove specific or assignable causes using RCA. They form a team, gather information, determine the basic condition that—if correct—prevents recurrence, and remove that condition from the system with a corrective action. Organizations can only remove common causes from the system by an action of management.

What exactly is an action of management? How could a diagnostic approach so important to improving complex systems be so vaguely described? This chapter provides the answer through two basic approaches to diagnose common causes based on the number of events, occurrences, and errors in the study. These include the following:

- Small, multiple event (three to 20 events)
- Large, multiple event (more than 20 events)

Each approach examines occurrences for common causes (shared local or global root causes) and common causes (variation causing normal problems within the system). Since these approaches all result in the removal of root causes from the system, common cause analysis is a form of RCA.

### Small, multiple-event common-cause analysis

Common-cause analysis is an RCA activity defined as any structured problem-solving technique that results in a corrective action to prevent the recurrence of an event. A small, multiple-event common-cause analysis simultaneously examines a few RCA events to determine whether the local system problems (the individual root causes) could be representative of larger, global systems problems.

If there are only two (or maybe three in some cases) events, we recommend you use a direct derivation technique. List the root causes of each event and answer the following basic commonality questions (two tests):

- Are the root causes of each event similar such that the incidents could be the result of a more global system problem?
- Are the root causes of each event dissimilar, but there exists a system failure mode that could result in the events?

If the root causes of event are radically different, there is less likelihood that there is a common cause. For an example, consider two events that occurred in the same labor and delivery unit. Both events resulted in hyper-stimulation of the mother's uterus because of human error in the administration of Pitocin®. In the first case, the nurse made a cognitive decision-making error in determining the dose because of the complexity in the protocol. In the second case, a different nurse made a simple slip error in determining the dose because of an inadequate mental state after returning to work after a long absence. Both occurrences have identical consequences and occur close together in time. Are the two occurrences the result of a common cause?

The first test indicates that they are not the result of a common cause. Although identical in consequence, the two occurrences have radically different causes: one is a process problem and the other is a human error that is, at worst case, representative of an organizational problem. This makes a common cause less likely.

Now consider the second test. Is there a common failure in the system that could result in both root causes even though the root causes are different? For example, consider two cases that occurred in an infusion center during patient identification: In the first case, a nurse experienced a simple lapse error and did not positively identify the patient. Had the nurse identified the patient by comparing the controlling document to the patient identification bracelet, he would have noticed that an error had occurred and the treatment was intended for another patient. In the second case, another nurse in the same infusion center consciously shortcut patient identification, allowing the wrong treatment on the patient. Are the two occurrences the result of a common cause?

In this case yes. Simple slip/lapse errors and noncompliance share a possible cause: poor accountability. People with poor accountability pay less attention to tasks and thereby make more slip/lapse errors.

People with poor accountability also are less compliant, thereby resulting in more work-rule violations. Although not seen in these two examples, people with poor accountability are also less likely to seek help when unsure and are less conservative in their own decision-making. The shared possible cause in this case—poor accountability—was confirmed and demonstrated as substandard when compared to other nursing units. The actual common cause was even deeper in the failure scenario. Poor supervisory skills in nursing leaders led to poor accountability, which in turn led to the high human error rate in nursing.

### Stream analysis

If there are more than two RCAs (three to 20 cases), an organization will obtain best results by using a structured technique to simplify the problem solving and show the results. Stream analysis and change analysis are best for this purpose.

Stream analysis in this application is similar to the affinity diagram—a basic quality tool—and the dendrogram (from the Greek "tree-picture"). A stream analysis shows several failure scenarios as text boxes (each text box representing a causative condition in the system) connected with arrows to indicate a cause-and-effect relationship. A schematic of a stream analysis is shown in Figure 10.2.

Figure 10.2 **An Example Stream Analysis Using Four Common Streams**

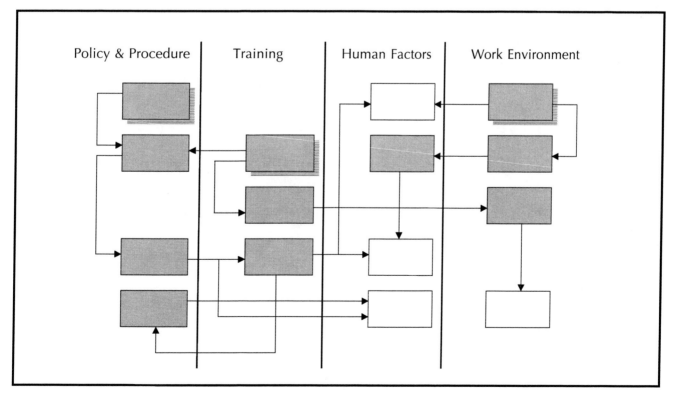

Interpreting a stream analysis is very simple. A box with only arrows coming in (no arrows out) is an observed problem. Fix these with remedial corrective action. A box with only arrows coming out (no arrows in) is a root cause. Fix these with corrective actions to prevent recurrence. Boxes with arrows in and arrows out are intermediate failure modes in the system. Only fix these when the condition is so high-risk/substandard that there is a strong need to accelerate the effects of the corrective actions to prevent recurrence. In the schematic in Figure 10.2, there are three root causes, seven intermediate failure modes, and four effects.

To perform the analysis, start with the RCAs. Review each analysis to determine the problems (effects), the failure modes in the system, and the root causes. Write each on a yellow sticky note and place the notes on a large sheet of paper. Arrange the notes so that the causes are in the center, the failure modes are in a belt surrounding the problems, and the root causes are in the outermost belt surrounding the intermediate failure modes. In this construction, the cause-and-effect arrows should generally point to the center. This is a dendrogram.

To make this a stream analysis, form all similar notes into columns based on which portion of the system failed to produce the event. For example, all of the policy and procedure tabs are in one column and all of the education and training notes are in another column. The cause-and-effect arrows should then travel in all directions. For further information on this process, we suggest you read *Stream Analysis* by Dr. Jerry Porras, Addison and Wesley Publishing Company (1994).

Now analyze for common cause using the following tests:

- Are the root causes of each event similar such that the events could be the result of a more global system problem?
- Are the root causes of each event dissimilar, but there exists a system failure mode that could result in the events?

Only the analysis is greatly simplified by the graphical depiction of the failure scenarios. If the failure scenarios overlap, the first test is positive. If the scenarios do not overlap, then examine the root causes using the second test.

## Change analysis

Change analysis is also a well-known basic RCA technique. However, in this application, the change analysis is simultaneously performed on the root causes, the failure modes, and the effects of several cases. Changes analysis could also be called difference analysis because the technique examines for similarity and difference between several conditions.

Place each root cause, failure mode, and effect in the rows of the table. Enter the information from each case in the columns, corresponding to the applicable row. Now examine the causes for commonality at the failure-mode and root cause levels. Use the very same two tests listed above to determine common cause.

Shannon Sayles, RN, MS, manager of performance improvement at Sentara Health Care in Norfolk, VA, performed an excellent example of this technique as a common-cause analysis. Her team examined an unexplained increase in the number of sedative reversal agents administered during a six-week period. The team used the change/difference analysis to evaluate for common cause since there were no clear commonalities in the 10 cases.

First the team examined the usual suspects. There was little or no commonality in the drug used, the surgical procedure, the surgeon, nurse, nursing unit, etc. The team dug a little deeper; there was little or no commonality in patient condition, patient selection, timing of doses, the location of dose administration (recovery v. floor), etc. Then some common themes emerged. The patients tended to be smaller than average, but not unusually small. The patients tended to be older, but not unusually old. The initial doses tended to be larger, but not out of the acceptable range, and most patients were not on supplemental oxygen. A solution then emerged: the renal clearance tended to be poor. Renal clearance, combined with the small patient size, large first dose, and poor oxygenation, provided enough variation in the system (all in the adverse direction) to expose the common causes. The protocol was revised to better account for these factors.

The case is an excellent success story because the analysis occurred at an outstanding hospital that is aggressively working to further improve performance. It also identified the system problem and corrected it using less-significant cases. Not one of the 10 cases was significant enough in itself to prompt an RCA. This is a good testament to the use of precursor events.

## Large, multiple-event common-cause analysis

As stated previously, common-cause analysis is an RCA activity, defined as any structured problem-solving technique that results in a corrective action to prevent recurrence of an event. A large, multiple-event common -cause analysis examines the aggregate effects of several typically less significant occurrences. In this instance, the organization should have taken remedial corrective actions for each occurrence. The common cause analysis then identifies more fundamental causes of the events as a set, investigates directly to determine root causes, and identifies corrective actions for those root causes.

The first step in performing a large, multiple-event common-cause analysis is to select the common-cause analysis data set. Often, this is already done when hospital managers provide the cause analysis team with a written charter defining the scope of the problem. Sometimes the scope is very specific: analyze all of the moderate sedation occurrences for the last two years and provide recommendations that will reduce the error rate by 80% in two years. Other scopes are less detailed, such as, "Make sure that we never have another retained foreign object during a surgical procedure."

Construct a spreadsheet or database to capture the data. Include as a minimum the following dimensions:

- Incident report number
- Occurrence description
- Condition or inappropriate action description
- Organization causing the inappropriate action
- Process controlling the action
- Activity in progress at the time the action occurs
- Causal factor information

Then analyze each occurrence in the data set for conditions and inappropriate actions. Capture applicable information as codes in the spreadsheet or database for each condition/inappropriate action. Code conditions by description, organization, process, and causal factor. Code an inappropriate action in all dimensions. Do not reinvestigate the event. Use the information provided to you and your knowledge of the organization/process to make reasonable conclusions based on available facts.

Now analyze the data for common causes. This is done using a Pareto chart as a visual guide to graphically summarize the relative importance of the difference between groups of data. Use the spreadsheet to refresh the analysts on specific details. Common causes are identified by their symptom pattern. Examine the combinations of organization, process, activity, and cause for the symptom patterns of known common causes. Capture these possible common causes for more analysis.

Poor communication between two organizations is a classical example of a common cause. The symptom pattern should include the two affected organizations, be spread among several processes and activities, have external causal factors of "inadequate interface among organizations [an organizational and programmatic failure mode], and have human error failure modes such as "wrong assumptions" or "misinterpretation of information."

Now form a theory that explains why this symptom pattern is present in the system. The theory should be an extension of the existing causal factor information. For our simple communication example, the causal factors might point to a poorly defined communication channel (the method of communication such as a telephone or digital pager.) A complete theory describes both the problem (communications) and the possible cause (the communication channel).

Confirm that the theory is correct before taking action. PII's experience in 10 years of common cause analysis has shown that 50% of the theories are not true common causes. Some theories are merely the result of bias in the RCAs or bias in the symptom pattern recognition. Other theories represent true conditions the system, but the condition is not substandard/cost-effective to correct.

Katherine Jones, PharmD, patient safety and investigative drug pharmacist at Memorial Health University Hospital in Savannah, GA, recently performed an excellent example of a large, multiple-event common-cause analysis. Her team performed a common-cause analysis of medication process occurrences for an 18-month period. They examined 164 incident reports, resulting in 200 inappropriate actions coded into a spreadsheet. The team also produced Pareto charts. The multidimensional analysis resulted in 10 common-cause theories.

## Apparent-cause analysis

PII, in performing common-cause analyses in health care, has found that most incident reports do not have sufficient information to determine an inappropriate action leading to the occurrence. As a result, the more successful common-cause analyses are based on the more significant occurrences that received an RCA. The majority of the incident reports do not contribute to system improvement. You will need apparent-cause analysis to perform common-cause analysis in your incident reporting system.

Apparent-cause analysis is an inexpensive and quick way to leverage system improvement information from less-significant occurrences. Health care has a consistent idea of what RCA means. There is, however, little consistency in the use of the term "apparent cause." Some hospitals use the words entered on the incident report in the block, "Why did this happen," as the apparent cause. A few hospitals actually perform an abbreviated cause analysis called "apparent cause." Most hospitals do not have an apparent cause analysis feature in their incident-reporting systems; they either do an RCA or nothing at all.

To PII, apparent-cause analysis is a specific cause-analysis activity. Apparent-cause analysis is the logical conclusion of what and why it happened, based on facts readily available. In practice, an apparent cause analysis captures one or two inappropriate actions—with failure modes—that led to the occurrence.

An RCA may require a team of five people working for 45 days; an apparent-cause analysis only requires one person working for one day. An RCA has two or three root cause conditions, each with a corrective action to prevent recurrence, written in a 10-page report along with the supporting facts and an event and casual factor chart. A good apparent cause analysis fits on one page and avoids sweeping corrective actions to prevent recurrence, concentrating instead on small improvements.

### When should organizations perform apparent cause?

Significant events, including sentinel events, require an RCA. However, the less significant occurrences only require remedial corrective actions for any problems that the organization identifies on the occurrence report. This makes apparent-cause analysis a choice by the hospital to invest in system improvement. Choose the best opportunities to improve your health care delivery system. The best opportunities are usually near-miss or precursor events of actual sentinel events. (See Chapter 9 for an explanation of how standard screening criteria for root cause and apparent-cause analysis is one of the 25 critical success factors of effective programs.) Think of the near-misses that you would like to investigate as RCAs, but you do not have the staff or the time or the resources to conduct them. This is exactly the purpose that apparent cause analysis is intended to fulfill.

Base your RCA and apparent-cause analysis projects on the significance of the individual occurrence. In the long-term, you should adjust the significance screening criteria to optimize the learning effectiveness of the incident-reporting system, also called the corrective action process). The optimal ratio of RCA to apparent cause analysis projects is 1:10. So if you performed eight RCAs last year, your goal in apparent cause analysis should be 80 per year. Remember that each apparent cause analysis is only eight staff hours while each RCA represents hundreds of staff hours.

### How to do apparent cause analysis

A good apparent cause analysis has the following three productive results for a hospital:

- It examines and solves a problem of some significance
- It examines a system problem and confirms it as not significant (and therefore doesn't require an RCA)
- It captures inappropriate actions with causal factors for use later in a common cause analysis

Begin your apparent cause analysis with the end in mind. Your apparent cause analysis will fit on one page with five basic elements

- A one-paragraph description of the occurrence.

- A one-paragraph explanation, based on objective evidence that confirms that the occurrence was not significant in consequence or widespread in extent of condition. If you cannot confirm, you should deem the occurrence as significant and escalate the apparent cause analysis to an RCA.

- The remedial corrective actions for any problems are listed on the incident report or discovered in the analysis.

- A one-paragraph (newspaper-style construction with who, what, when, why, and how) description of the cause(s) based on available facts.

- The corrective actions to prevent recurrence for the few cases where a low-risk and cost-effective solution is clearly available.

Send one person to investigate the occurrence using information collection methods similar to RCA, but scaled down in time and formality. Gather facts in the case by reviewing the medical record, talking to the people involved, and reviewing the work environment. Then assemble the facts into the apparent-cause analysis. Do not just assign causal-factor codes to inappropriate actions. Explain the occurrence without the use of buzzwords or jargon so an independent cause analyst could understand the occurrence and assign causal factor codes in any diagnostic system.

To get started in apparent-cause analysis you need to follow these three steps:

- Develop significance criteria to screen each incident report for apparent cause opportunities.

- Educate your staff on your approach to apparent-cause analysis, otherwise they will hurriedly perform poor RCA

- Develop a standard report format to simplify the analysis

These three easy steps will enable your hospital to learn from less significant occurrences in real-time and provide for an effective common-cause analysis program (all the effectiveness of the entire RCA program with one-tenth the resources) in the long-term.

## Summary

Performing an effective RCA is an important part of the patient safety movement. But to truly create an effective program that will prevent the recurrence of events, it's important that health care organizations consider the next step of the process: common-cause analysis.

# CHAPTER 11

## Help! What's With All These Terms?

# CHAPTER 11

# Help! What's With All These Terms?

This section includes definitions of important terms used throughout this book and detailed discussion of key concepts important to performance improvement (PI) and root cause analysis (RCA). For the reader's convenience, we've provided a list below of the terms and concepts covered in this section.

## Occurrence/event terminology

- Consequence
- Event (also referred to as an adverse event, terminal event, and occurrence)
- Inappropriate action (human error)
- Problem identification/reporting
- Sentinel event
- Symptom

## Cause-analysis terminology

- Apparent cause
- Apparent-cause analysis
- Causal factor
- Common cause
- Common-cause analysis
- Contributing cause
- Evidence matrix
- Failure mode or failure mechanism
- Failure scenario

- Qualification, Validation, and Verification (QV&V)
- Refuting evidence
- Root cause
- Root cause analysis
- Root solution
- Substandard performance
- Supporting evidence
- Technology-based cause analysis, technology-based failure modes
- Three-meeting model

## Transportability terminology

- Extent of condition
- Generic implications

## Recommendation/corrective action terminology

- Corrective action to prevent recurrence (CATPR)
- Interim corrective action (compensatory action)
- Remedial corrective action

## Performance improvement and other terminology

- Key activity
- Organization
- Process
- PII's Performance Pyramid
- Culture and performance

### *Occurrence/event terminology*

**Consequence**: The adverse result of an event that is often expressed in terms of safety (such as injury), financial loss (such as equipment damage or production loss), environmental impact (such as chemical spill or radiological exposure), and image (such as customer satisfaction).

**Event** (also referred to as an adverse event, terminal event, or occurrence): A happening or occurrence of undesired consequences. All events happen for a reason. People design and implement systems and then carry out the majority of actions within a system or process. Therefore, organizations must analyze events in terms of the actions people took that resulted in the undesired incident.

**Inappropriate action**: A euphemism for human error. Some inappropriate actions do not result in significant consequences while others create an undesired or unwanted consequence.

In the first case, an inappropriate action occurs when the individual clearly does not meet a performance expectation or standard, but there is no significant adverse consequence. An example is the case of individuals who do not wash their hands before performing a treatment or examination of a patient. Even if there was no negative impact to the patient, the action (of not washing their hands) was inappropriate. Another example is a phlebotomist who does not meet the hospital's policy of using two independent means of patient identification (such as patient name and birth date), but relies on the patient's room number. Even if the blood sample was drawn from the correct patient, there is still an inappropriate action because the phlebotomist did not use the hospital's policy for patient identification techniques.

Other inappropriate actions result in undesired or unwanted consequences regardless of the performance expectations. Often these inappropriate actions are learning moments for the individual and the organization. An example is improper use of a new piece of equipment that results in an unwanted expectation. Once the employee understands the correct use, the manager can develop a performance expectation. Another example involves surgeons who mistakenly operate on the wrong site because they failed to mark the correct location in accordance with hospital policy.

Humans are susceptible to the following basic types of inappropriate actions or human errors:

- Skill-based
- Rule-based
- Knowledge-based

## Skill-based errors

A skill-based error occurs when an individual commits a slip or lapse while performing routine actions in a familiar environment and they are functioning by habit or reflex with very little conscious thought.

The characteristics of skill-based errors include

- an unintentional slip or lapse when performing a familiar task
- a correct intention, but inappropriate action
- an error made by skilled personnel who are experts or well-practiced in the task
- an unintentional deviation from a planned or routine action

Typical error probabilities for errors during skill-based performance are approximately 0.1%-0.3%

## Rule-based errors

When individuals perform in a "rule-based" mode, they make conscious decisions about activities that they are familiar with, understand, and have experience performing. A rule-based error occurs if they misapply the rule because of a wrong assumption, misinterpretation of information, or incomplete information. Rule-based errors are also occur when an individual makes a conscious decision not to follow a rule or standard.

Rule-based errors

- occur during conscious decision-making tasks in which the individual is trained and experienced
- result when a rule from training, experience, or a procedure that is known to the individual is misapplied or consciously not followed (rule noncompliance)

Typical error probabilities for rule-based errors during performance are approximately 1.0%–3.0%

## Knowledge-based errors

When individuals perform in a "knowledge-based" mode, they make conscious decisions as in "rule-based" performance. However, in knowledge-based performance they are not trained or familiar with the task or activity, nor are they experienced in the task. But in trying to make a good decision their attention level is very high. They are thinking hard about the best course of action. If they commit a knowledge-based error it is usually because they do not have adequate training or experience in the task. Knowledge-based errors may also occur because "you don't know what you don't know."

The characteristics of knowledge-based errors include

- conscious decision-making tasks performed by an untrained or inexperienced individual
- a lack of contingency plans or preformed solutions for the problem
- an analytical or logical thought processing because the individual doesn't know of a specific "rule" to follow (even if one exists)

Typical error probabilities for knowledge-based errors during performance are approximately 10%-30%.

Understanding different error types is very important for an investigator since the causes of skill-based, rule-based, and knowledge-based inappropriate actions are unique from each other and therefore the corrective actions are dependent on the error type experienced

**Problem identification or problem reporting**: The act of reporting an event or occurrence to the organization. A hospital will often develop an electronic, manual/telephone reporting system that is available to all employees for the purposes of reporting issues or occurrences when they happen.

**Sentinel event**: A special term that the Joint Commission on Accreditation of Healthcare Organizations (JCAHO) defines in its *Comprehensive Accreditation Manual for Hospitals* (CAMH) as "an unexpected occurrence involving death or serious physical or psychological injury, or the risk thereof." Serious injury specifically includes loss of limb or function. The phrase, "or the risk thereof" includes any process variation for which a recurrence would carry a significant chance of a serious adverse outcome. Such events are called 'sentinel' because they signal the need for immediate investigation and response."

The following are examples of sentinel events that are voluntarily reportable under the JCAHO's Sentinel Event Policy, according to the CAMH:

- Any patient death, paralysis, coma, or other major permanent loss of function associated with a medication error

- Any suicide of a patient in a setting where the patient is housed around-the-clock, including suicides following elopement from such a setting

- Any elopement (i.e., unauthorized departure) of a patient from an around-the-clock care setting resulting in a temporally related death (suicide or homicide) or major permanent loss of function

- Any procedure on the wrong patient, wrong side of the body, or wrong organ.

- Any intrapartum (related to the birth process) maternal death

- Any perinatal death unrelated to a congenital condition in an infant having a birth weight greater than 2,500 grams

- Assault, homicide, or other crime resulting in patient death or major permanent loss of function

- A patient fall that results in death or major permanent loss of function as a direct result of the injuries sustained in the fall

- Hemolytic transfusion reaction involving major blood group incompatibilities

The CAMH lists the following examples of events that are not reportable to the JCAHO:

- Any near-miss

- Full return of limb or bodily function to the same level as prior to the adverse event by discharge or within two weeks of the initial loss of said function

- Any sentinel event that has not affected a recipient of care (patient, client, resident)

- Medication errors that do not result in death or major permanent loss of function

- Suicide other than in an around-the-clock care setting or following elopement from such a setting

- A death or loss of function following a discharge "against medical advice"

- Unsuccessful suicide attempts

- Unintentionally retained foreign body without major permanent loss of function

- Minor degrees of hemolysis with no clinical sequelae

**Symptom**: Any circumstance or condition that accompanies an event and is indicative of that event occurrence. Symptoms are typically observed and captured for use as information in identifying failure modes.

### Cause-analysis terminology

**Apparent cause**: A logical assumption of reason based on the available facts in the event.

**Apparent-cause analysis**: A limited investigation of an event that is often performed instead of RCA for less significant events. Apparent-cause analysis is a process to identify remedial corrective actions and to identify information necessary to support future common-cause analysis. Corrective action(s) to prevent recurrence are strongly discouraged when an organization only performs an apparent-cause analysis because the true root causes are not known with any confidence.

**Causal factor**: A condition in the system that shapes an outcome. Causal factors begin to answer the question "Why did this occur?" Typically, one or more causal factors acts to result in an observed failure mode (see definition for **failure mode or failure scenario**).

Fire is a good example for illustrating causal factors v. failure modes. A recent issue raised by the JCAHO in its *Sentinel Event Alert* in June 2003 is surgical room fires. A fire is a failure mode. Three causal factors combine to result in fire: heat, fuel, and oxygen. Causal factors are the ingredients in a recipe for a failure mode.

Because causal factors describe why something occurred, at some point in an investigation one or more causal factors become the root cause(s). A root cause is a very special causal factor. So, following our example, are the causal factors of heat, fuel, and oxygen the root causes of a surgical fire? No. Organizations must answer the question "How did we not appropriately control these causal factors that allowed the fire to occur?" The answer to this question may identify human performance or process issues and the associated causal factors at some point become the root cause(s).

**Common cause:** A statement of a condition that is responsible for many past events. Common causes may be local in nature (i.e., affecting specific areas within the organization) or global in nature (i.e., affecting most of the organization and transcending multiple work processes).

**Common-cause analysis**: An RCA activity that examines the aggregate effects of several, typically less significant events. Each event should already have received remedial corrective actions. The common-cause analysis identifies more fundamental causes of the events as a group, investigates directly to determine root causes, and identifies corrective actions for root causes.

**Contributing cause**: A causal factor that, if corrected, would not prevent recurrence of the condition but is significant enough to fix. Contributing causes often result in future unwanted events if left unaddressed.

**Evidence matrix**: A method the root cause investigator uses to organize supporting and refuting evidence against failure modes or other items of interest during an investigation. The evidence matrix is a very helpful tool when performing information Qualification, Validation, and Verification. (See entry for Qualification, validation, and verification.)

**Failure mode or failure mechanism**: An observed condition or symptom of a failure or the manner in which a failure evidences itself. The failure mode is the answer to the question, "How did this inappropriate action (which in part led to the event of interest) occur?"

A failure mode is a unique combination of conditions that come together to form that effect. Failure modes are sometimes confused with causal factors. A causal factor is a condition in the system that shapes an outcome. Failure modes are how words, where causal factors are why words. Each failure mode has a recipe and the ingredients are causal factors.

For example, a commonly seen failure mode in health care is "shortcuts evoked," which describes a situation in which individuals make a conscious decision not to follow a policy or procedure, such as not to wash their hands between treating patients. Three causal factors typically lead to shortcuts evoked: a perceived burden (i.e., it takes some unnecessary time to walk to the sink and wash my hands), poor coworker coaching culture (i.e., coworkers don't hold each other accountable to the handwashing standard), and low perceived risk of not washing (i.e., there is a low risk that something bad will happen to the patient or myself if I don't wash my hands.)

## Failure mode charts

If investigators know all possible failure modes, they are more likely to identify the specific characteristics of the event and have a higher likelihood of determining the true root cause(s). Many use failure mode charts, which describe all possible failure modes of the issue under investigation. A well-designed failure mode chart is mutually exclusive and collectively exhaustive. That is, each failure mode in the chart describes a unique condition (mutually exclusive of the others) and all the failure modes taken together describe all possible failure mechanisms (collectively exhaustive.)

For example, a bolt on your automobile or on a piece of equipment at your home fails in one of four possible failure modes: overload (too much force causes it to break), corrosion (it rusts to the point of failure), embrittlement (the metal fails at the grains of the material because of the environment in which it was manufactured or operated), and fatigue (the metal fails because of cyclic stresses).

## Human failure modes

People fail in a finite number of failure modes. Performance Improvement International (PII) has developed a failure mode chart for humans (called the Human Error/Inappropriate Action Chart) describing 28 failure modes for individuals. This chart includes these failure modes: wrong assumptions, inadequate motivation, shortcuts evoked, and overconfidence. (See the Appendix for the failure mode chart for humans.)

## Organizational and programmatic failure modes

Organizations and processes also fail in specific ways. PII's Organizational and Programmatic Diagnostic Chart (see the Appendix for the chart) describes the 18 that ways organizations and programs fail. Failure modes on this chart include inadequate interface among organizations, insufficient programmatic detail, and excessive implementation requirements.

## Executive management failure modes

Management and leadership teams are also susceptible to distinct failure modes. PII's *Executive Management Failure Mode Chart* defines 30 specific failure modes for management teams, including, "vague or unclear expectations," "unawareness of regulatory implications," "inadequate successor planning," and "inadequate accountability system." (See the Appendix for the *Executive Management Failure Mode Chart.*)

**Failure scenario**: A sequence of events that begins with the root cause and ends with the observed failure. A failure scenario is a narrative story that describes the sequence of events. In effect, it is a stream of causal factors from the root cause, passing through the failure mode, and ending at the observed event.

**Qualification, Validation, and Verification (QV&V)**: A logical thought process used to determine whether a piece of information is factual. Organizations should only use facts to determine failure modes, failure scenario, root cause(s) and corrective action(s) during an RCA.

The QV&V process consists of three steps: Qualification, Validation, and Verification. If each test is satisfied, the organization can consider a piece of information "factual" for the purposes of the root cause investigation. Qualification is the credibility of the information source. Validation is the sensibility of the information from the investigator's perspective. Verification is corroboration of the story with other information from an independent, qualified source. The best method of verification is the "rule of two": two pieces of independent information comprise a fact.

**Qualification** is a test of the information source. Does the organization believe the source to be reliable and credible based on the accuracy and completeness of past information? Is this person the appropriate source to provide the information? For example, a nurse manager should be a qualified source to provide information related to nursing policies and procedures.

**Validation** is an internal test on the information accuracy and completeness. Internal refers to the individual conducting the investigation. Does the information make sense to the investigator? Is the information consistent with other data available to the investigator? For example, if an individual described an event that was logical and consistent with other evidence, and makes sense to the investigator, the explanation would satisfy the validation test.

**Verification** is an independent test of the information's accuracy and completeness. Independent refers to the source. Can a second, qualified source corroborate the information? For example, if an employee indicated that he did not believe the hospital's inservice education program adequately prepared or qualified him to perform a task and other individuals in that work group voiced similar concerns, it would satisfy the verification test.

*Qualification* and *validation* are relatively simple and usually only require a few seconds of mental thought by the investigator. *Verification* is more time consuming, but is necessary when the information is key to the investigation, when either the qualification or validation tests fail, or when new information becomes available that brings into question the validity of other information or facts.

**Refuting evidence:** Information that does not support a particular conclusion or failure mode. Comparing supporting evidence and refuting evidence is part of the QV&V process.

**Root cause:** The most basic condition that, if corrected, prevents recurrence of the failure. To be considered a root cause, a causal factor must pass the following tests:

1. The condition has a proven cause-and-effect relationship. If the hospital removes the condition from the system, it will prevent the occurrence and have no harmful side effects.

2. The condition is within management's control to correct.

3. The condition is cost-effective to correct.

If all three conditions are satisfied, then the organization should consider the identified condition a "root cause." If any condition is not satisfied, then the organization needs to conduct additional analysis to identify the true root cause(s).

Because of the 'defense-in-depth" concept of using multiple process barriers in complex, higher-risk industries, the chance of a single condition being responsible for a significant adverse event is very low. Typically there are multiple root causes and therefore multiple areas to improve. Based on more than 5,000 root cause investigations conducted by PII since the mid-1980s, the average number of root causes per significant event is approximately 2.8.

**Root cause analysis (RCA):** A structured problem-solving technique that results in one or more corrective actions to prevent recurrence of an event. Organizations should make sure that individuals who are specially trained in basic and advanced RCA techniques perform these activities.

RCA typically examines a single, significant occurrence; a set of similar occurrences (similar in consequence and/or in cause(s)); or an adverse trend in less-significant occurrences. The RCA process described in this book is composed of the following distinct steps:

1. Investigate the event or occurrence, that is define the problems, the inappropriate actions and the issues of interest. (See **Chapter 3,** "Investigate the Event.")

2. Collect and process data—sort out the facts using QV&V. (See **Chapter 4,** "Just the Facts, Please! Collecting Data and Information.")

3. Identify the failure modes—also called failure mechanisms. (See **Chapter 5,** "How to Identify the Failure Modes.")

4. Construct failure scenario(s)—a sequence of events from root cause(s) to observed problems (See **Chapter 6,** "Develop the Failure Scenario[s].)

5. Develop root solutions—benchmark your results to organization's experience, your industry's experience, and if appropriate, experience in other industries and then develop root cause(s) and associated corrective actions to prevent recurrence. (See **Chapter 7,** "Develop Root Solutions.")

6. Monitor the effectiveness—determine whether the organization has implemented corrective actions and whether they are effective. (See **Chapter 8,** "Monitor for Effectiveness—The Last Step.")

**Root solution**: The pairing of a root cause(s) and the associated corrective actions to prevent recurrence. The real goal of a root cause investigation is to determine the root solution—not just the root cause.

**Substandard performance**: Actions that don't meet generally accepted practices, conditions, or established standards. Only substandard organizational and programmatic, human factor, work environment, and management failure modes can be root causes. If the standard is met, the system is not deficient and the cause of the occurrence is an isolated human error or equipment failure.

**Supporting evidence**: Information that supports a particular conclusion or failure mode. Comparing supporting evidence and refuting evidence is part of the QV&V process.

**Technology-based cause analysis and technology-based failure modes**: Cause analysis that is based on proven methodologies and comprehensive listings of failure modes. A technology-based approach to RCA, such as the one recommended by these authors, ensures that the organization considers all known failure mechanisms and provides a rigorous process for uncovering those it doesn't know.

**Three-meeting model**: An effective structure used to facilitate the completion of the six steps in the root cause investigation process. The model allows an experienced root cause investigator to conduct the investigation in an efficient manner by bringing the appropriate people together during an RCA without wasting people's time in meetings they need not attend.

### Transportability terminology

**Extent of condition:** The transportability of the symptoms. Once an organization identifies an event, it must consider the extent of condition (i.e., Where else could this type of problem exist?) Extent of condition is typically addressed early in the cause analysis by applying remedial corrective actions to similarly affected areas.

For example, assume a nurse incorrectly programs an infusion pump, resulting in an improper administration of medication. Upon discovery, it appears the nurse does not fully understand how to properly program the pump. The extent of condition question would consider, "What other pumps has the nurse programmed recently?" Perhaps she had problems in the past that were not discovered. The organization must take appropriate remedial corrective actions for the identified deficiencies.

**Generic implications:** Transportability of the cause. Once an event is understood through RCA, there is a question of what is the impact on the system or organization, which is, "If this is the cause, what does this mean to us?" Generic implications are typically addressed late in the cause analysis (after the event is understood) by applying appropriate corrective actions to similarly affected areas and by carrying out compensatory actions.

For example, assume once again that a nurse incorrectly programs an infusion pump, resulting in a misadministration of medication. The RCA reveals that the inservice education session did not adequately address all the information necessary to reliably program the pump. The generic implications question would address all affected nurses and why the inservice process failed to adequately train the staff.

### Recommendation/corrective action terminology

**Corrective action to prevent recurrence (CATPR):** An action taken to prevent recurrence of the undesirable event by eliminating the root cause(s). CATPRs are also called preventive actions. Recall that a root cause is the most fundamental causal factor that, if corrected, prevents recurrence of the event. So in effect, a root cause is the causal factor associated with a CATPR. In fact, you cannot define root cause and CATPR independent of one another.

A CATPR must meet three conditions: it must address the identified root cause, it must be cost-effective, and it must be within the capability of management to implement in a reasonable time frame.

**Interim corrective action:** A short-term action designed to reduce risk of recurrence during the implementation of longer-term corrective actions to prevent recurrence. Interim corrective actions are also called compensatory actions.

For example, if individuals commit an inappropriate action due to lack of knowledge or competency, supervisors should not assign them that task as an interim corrective action until they receive adequate training.

**Remedial corrective action:** An action designed to restore a condition or a situation to the desired state. Remedial corrective actions are typically carried out immediately after problem discovery and are intended to minimize immediate risk. Organizations can implement remedial corrective actions independent of the root cause(s). These actions are also called remedial actions.

For example, if a nurse administered a medication to the wrong patient, remedial actions would probably include notification to the appropriate physician(s), administering the proper medication to the patient who did not receive it, responding in an appropriate manner to the patient who received the wrong medication, and initiating an occurrence or problem report per hospital policy.

### Performance improvement and other terminology

**Key activity:** A specific function of a process that is typically executed by a single organization or professional group. For example, a physician performs many key activities as part of patient care, such as conducting a history and physical, ordering tests or medications, and performing procedures.

**Organization:** A group of people with similar knowledge and skills assigned to execute specific functions. In a hospital the various departments are examples of an organization. For instance, pharmacy, radiology, emergency department, and a medical/surgical floor all meet the definition of an organization. Because of the matrix-type organizational structure in a hospital, certain professional groups would also meet the definition of an organization, such as nursing.

**Process:** A series of actions (called key activities) that organizations specify to execute a function or to transform an input to a desired output.

For example, the delivery of medications to a patient is a process. The medication process contains several key activities, accomplished by different organizations or professional groups. These activities include the physician ordering the medication, the pharmacist dispensing the medication, and the nurse administering the medication.

## PII's Performance Pyramid

It is a generally accepted fact that the majority of significant adverse events in complex, higher-risk industries are caused by system issues, such as organizational breakdowns, programmatic deficiencies, process problems, or cultural weaknesses. Based on more than 5,000 root cause investigations in nuclear power production, aviation, manufacturing, and health care, we estimate that more than 85% of the root causes are associated with programmatic breakdowns, organizational deficiencies, or management issues. The figure on the next page illustrates this important concept.

In order to maximize performance in an organization, leaders must take two actions. First, through initiative, integrity, and involvement, they must create a culture that is conducive to excellence in human performance. Second, they must establish and maintain robust processes that are error tolerant, thereby preventing unwanted events due to a single human error. Supervisors must control their department's performance to the standards, expectations, and goals established by hospital leaders. Every individual in the organization must pay attention to detail, use good judgment, maintain an appropriate mental state, be committed to the desired outcomes, and develop their knowledge and skills.

Having said this, what types of problems or issues does an organization face? The Performance Pyramid provides the answer: individual performance issues, localized organizational or programmatic issues, and global issues. Each is shown in the figure below and discussed in more detail in the following paragraphs.

### Individual performance issues

Some problems are truly individual performance issues. Individuals may commit inappropriate actions because of their own mental state, not related to or influenced by the organization's culture or its processes. For example, imagine employees who have personal problems (financial, health, marital, etc.) that affect their mental state while at work. It is easy to imagine them experiencing errors that result in an unwanted event. In complex, high-risk industries, events caused by isolated, individual performance problems constitute a small percentage of the population (less than 15%).

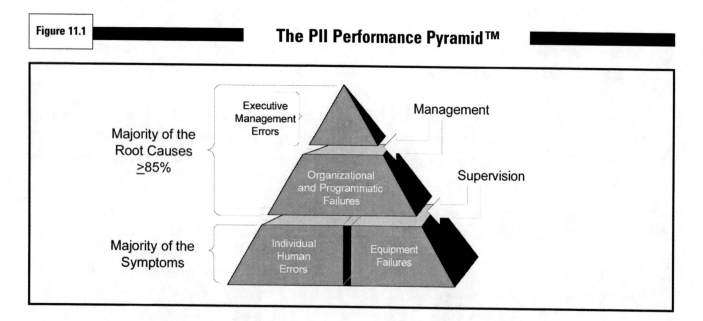

**Figure 11.1** **The PII Performance Pyramid™**

Figure 11.2 **Three Types of Problems in an Organization**

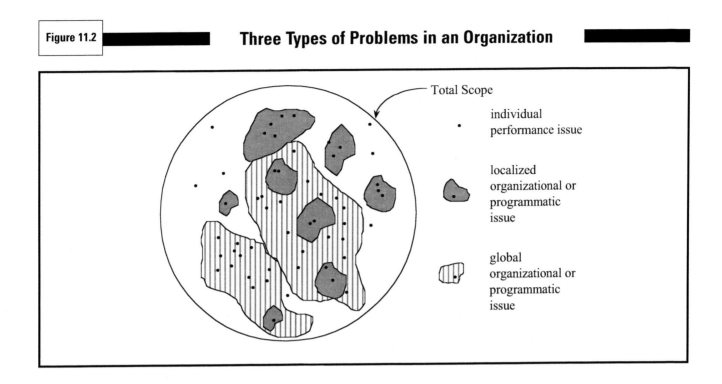

## Organizational and programmatic failures

The second type of problem encountered is called a localized organizational and programmatic (or process) failure. In this case, several events occur because of a common cause related to limited portions of the organization or limited to a specific process. For example, assume there are interface problems (called poor lateral integration) between two professional groups, such as nurses and physicians. These lateral integration problems might be due to a noncooperative culture, inadequate integration mechanisms, or poor communication skills and communication error prevention techniques. This localized issue will result in unwanted events when completing tasks that require good communication and coordination between the affected groups.

## Global issues

The third type of problem encountered is called a global issue, which affects large portions of the organization, usually transcends many processes or programs, and usually cultural in nature. Examples of global issues include widespread noncompliance with standards and policies, ineffective frontline supervision, poorly identified organizational vision, mission, and goals, weak strategic planning, poor cultivation of people in the organization, and low procedural quality.

Mature organizations have often identified and solved individual performance issues and localized issues. They are more apparent to the root cause investigators and managers. Global issues are harder to identify and solve but the benefits are huge to the organization—a rising tide affects all ships. Traditional RCA techniques are not very effective at the identification and solution of global issues. Common-cause analysis coupled with advanced RCA techniques is the most effective way to identify and solve these problems.

## Culture and performance

There is a well-known concept that "culture drives behaviors and behaviors determine outcomes." But how does culture really affect an organization's performance? What are the key characteristics of a high-performing culture? Can an organization qualitatively and quantitatively measure its culture and use it to predict its future performance? Let's begin to answer these important questions with an analogy.

Significant event rate (such as sentinel event rate in a hospital) is a measure of the safety performance of an organization just as the integrity of a building is measured by the condition of the space it protects from external elements. An organization's "culture" is analogous to the building's foundation. If it is strong, there is a greater likelihood that the organization's future performance or the building's future integrity will be strong. However, a building that has a good foundation can also have structural flaws in the walls or roof. Therefore, a building's foundation is only one of two factors on which the integrity of the building depends. The balance of the structure is the other factor. In a hospital these other "structural flaws" are evidenced by localized organizational or programmatic deficiencies. As the soundness of the foundation alone does not determine the integrity of the structure, the hospital's culture alone does not determine the level of safety performance.

But what is a "safe" culture? In general terms, a safe culture is one that promotes behaviors throughout the organization that result in safe, reliable, and productive performance. A safe culture exhibits five key characteristics as indicated in the following figure:

Strong missions and goals are very important to the health of an organization, and it's up to hospital leaders to establish and communicate these messages. The organization must also set behavior-based expectations and a work-prioritization system that are consistent with the mission. It must establish a system to track progress toward the goals, as well as assign responsibility through an accountability program.

All workers, supervisors, and managers should have a strong knowledge and skill base. Coworker coaching, pre-job briefings, reviews and requirements, training and qualification, and careful selection of the right workers for the right jobs are all important elements to maintaining a high level of knowledge and skills in the organization. While policies and procedures are very important, knowledge and skills are the last line of defense against unwanted events.

Lateral integration is defined as the mechanisms and culture that help interactions and communications among individuals, groups, and organizations. Lateral integration is made possible by a cooperative cul-

Figure 11.3 **Five Key Characteristics of Culture**

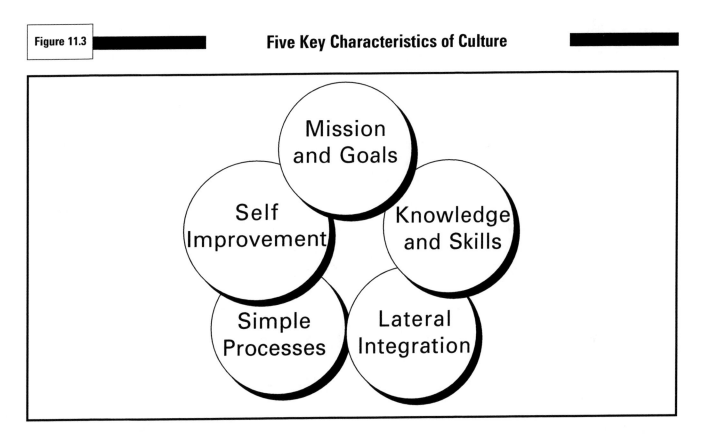

ture in addition to intergroup interface mechanisms, problem-solving coordination mechanisms, and task collaboration mechanisms. Department-to-department meetings, clearly defined responsibilities, authority, and accountability, and off-site activities to enhance trust between coworkers are all methods to ensure good lateral integration. Good lateral integration will decrease the rate of rule-based errors.

Overly complex processes can induce human error and inefficiency. High-performing organizations continually work to simplify work processes and programs. They keep administrative programs to a minimum; reduce unneeded regulatory commitments, verifications, or reviews; and encourage employees to develop multiple skills.

A self-improvement culture is the driving force to correct organizational and programmatic problems. Organizations should establish a performance monitoring and trending program, conduct root cause and common-cause analyses, take preventive measures, and encourage workers to report deficiencies and non-conformity.

### Characteristics of culture

Can organizations quantitatively measure their cultures and use them as predictors of future performance? The answer is yes. Managers can analyze the strength of each of the five key characteristics using employee surveys and validation interviews. Over the past 15 years, PII has used a "culture index" survey to accomplish the measurement. While the treatment of the measurement tool and the analysis of the data are beyond the scope of this book, a brief explanation follows.

Approximately 50 characteristics describe the five key characteristics of culture just presented. We evaluate these characteristics and use them to assign a score (from zero to four points) in each of the five key characteristics. Summed, the individual scores result in a culture index score of between zero and 20 points. Based on approximately 300 culture index determinations in all industries, an organization's future performance (e.g., safety, productivity) will improve if its culture index score is greater than or equal to 14 points. Those organizations that scored between 11 and 14 points remained relatively stable in performance unless they took actions to improve weaker areas. All of the organizations that had a Culture Index score of less than or equal to 11 points declined in future performance unless they took actions to remediate the weak areas.

But how do cultural deficiencies actually cause performance problems? Imagine if a cultural evaluation determined that your organization's key characteristic of lateral integration was weak. Lateral integration is associated with teamwork, trust, and communications in the organization. Therefore, if it is weak, then the organization would experience events due to miscommunication. The organization would have difficulty dealing with issues that transcend organizational or department boundaries or that requires cooperation and coordination from various professional groups.

# APPENDIX

- Personal statement
- Problem statement
- How to conduct effective interviews
- Interview form
- Event and Causal Factor Charting
- Change analysis
- Barrier analysis
- Barrier analysis worksheet—health care example
- Task analysis
- Stream analysis
- Selection and comparison of root cause analysis techniques
- Work environment factors (conditions inducing human error)
- Human factors (conditions inducing human error)
- Human error/ inappropriate action failure mode chart
- Organizational and programmatic diagnostic chart
- Executive management failure mode chart
- The top 12 high-risk behaviors causing sentinel events in health care
- The top 12 high-risk situations causing sentinel events in health care

## Personal statement

**Event description** _____

**Event date/time** _____

**Name** _____

**Position** _____

**Date/time statement completed** _____

In your own words, please describe what you saw, heard, felt, or thought before, during, and shortly after the event—provide as much information as possible. Please try to answer the following basic questions: When? Where? What? Who? How? How Many?

_____

_____

_____

_____

_____

_____

_____

_____

███████████████████  **Problem statement**  ███████████████████

**Steps to define the problem:**

1. In order to define the incident, first list the pertinent facts:

Who was involved (use titles, avoid names)?

_____

_____

What happened?

_____

_____

When did the problem occur?

_____

_____

How much/how many/or how long?

_____

_____

2. Gather this information into a single problem statement. Keep in mind that you want your problem statement to bound the analysis, to focus on what you actually know, to be precise, and to define a "problem" not a conclusion. (The problem statement should define symptoms, not present conclusions.)

**Initial problem statement:**

_____

_____

## How to conduct effective interviews

### Overview

Interviewing is one of the most powerful tools in conducting an event evaluation. Interviews should be fact finding and not fault finding. Two interviews are often necessary: the initial "on the scene" data collection and follow-up fill-in-the-gaps or confirmatory interviews. Drafting preliminary event and causal factor chart may be a helpful tool in preparing for the interview as it will help ensure all necessary information is obtained. However, initial "on-the-scene" interview and written statement may have to be conducted immediately to avoid loss of vital information or "group think" (convincing one another what's supposed to have happened) among the involved people.

Interviews should include individuals who are either directly or indirectly involved in the event or condition; including management personnel and personnel responsible for applicable training and procedure development. Particular attention should be given to lines of communication between supervisors and workers.

Information obtained in the interviews should be validated with physical data or independently verified through several interviews. If the interviewee does not respond adequately or shows a lack of knowledge in the area, the subject should be changed or the interview closed. Sometimes confirmatory interviews, especially with the interviewee's supervisor, are necessary to confirm facts from previous interviews.

Close the interview by summarizing the discussion to verify accuracy and to provide the interviewee an opportunity to fill in any additional information.

Because people tend to forget vital information quickly, initial interviews should be conducted as soon as possible after the event to be most effective in gathering accurate information; e.g. before they go home, during the shift in which the event happened or shortly thereafter.

### Preparation

Preparation for interviews is important, but prompt contact with participants and witnesses is also a concern. If possible interviews should be done within three days of the event. For personnel on shift, attempt to contact the individuals during the shift in which the event happened and seek management support to have the individuals hold-over when necessary.

## How to conduct effective interviews (cont.)

In preparing for the interview, RCA team members should consider the following:

- Why is the information being gathered?
- What type of information is expected from the interview?
- Has the event happened before?
- Are there any (known) outside pressures that could be a factor in the responses?
- Are there any circumstances that are likely to make the interviewees hostile or reluctant to speak freely?

All interviews require preparation no matter how simple the event appears to be. The interviewer should try to perform the following before beginning the interview:

- Construct a preliminary 'event and causal factors chart' to ensure that no major gaps exist in your initial understanding of the event.

- Develop a list of interviewees

- Make appointments for interviews with management liaisons.

- Schedule the interviews in the reverse order of involvement. Talk first to those who had the least involvement. The more you know about the subject before talking to those directly involved will stimulate better questions.

- Plan and write questions down ahead of time, this will provide direction for keeping the interview on track.

- Review procedures, drawings, and other work documents that were or should have been used in the event.

- Conduct one-on-one interviews because they are usually the most effective for initial data collection.

- Make sure interviews include an introduction, a questioning phase, and a closing phase.

## How to conduct effective interviews (cont.)

### Introduction phase

To orient the interviewees and put them at ease, keep the following guidelines in mind:

- Conduct the interview in a private and non-threatening environment.

- Start the conversation with an unrelated subject (ice-breaker) to put the interviewee at ease.

- Make simple changes,such as moving the location of the interview to a neutral location , because they may produce much more productive sessions.

- Present a clear statement of purpose for the interview. Explain why you are holding interviews and why you selected the interviewee.

- Explain that you will attempt to maintain confidentiality, if appropriate.

- Explain that you are trying to establish facts and are not there to place blame.

### Questioning phase

To obtain the interviewee's recollection of the event, consider the following:

- Spend more time listening (70%) than talking. Interrupt only if you do not understand. Expect silent pauses.
- Ask broad questions  first (10-15 minutes), then follow them up with specific questions (20-30 minutes).
- Keep questions short and simple. Let interviewees use their own words.
- Never use multiple-choice questions.
- Never argue.
- Be objective. Conduct the interview without any preassumptions.
- Use diagrams or drawings to help the interviewee. walk through his activity during the event..
- Minimize non-related conversation after the initial ice-breaker.

## How to conduct effective interviews (cont.)

- Take good notes. Tape recording is never recommended.
- Make sure interactions are professional and polite.
- Do not provide *Immunity* of any kind.

### Closing phase

As you end the interview, consider the following:

- Determine how the interviewee's behavior in the task of interest was influenced.

- Determine if the interviewee is aware of any changes related to the task of interest.

- Use broad questions , such as 'Can you tell me anything more?, at the end of the interview.'

- Decide whether another interview is necessary. Sometimes you will need to conduct multiple interviews. The first may consist solely of hearing the narrative. Arrange a second, more detailed interview if you have further questions.

## Interview form

Name(s): _____

Position(s): _____

Department(s): _____

Date and time of incident: _____

**Suggested interview questions:**

**When?**
When did the "event" occur: day, date, time, shift, and hours on shift?

Was it the first day of a long weekend, holiday?

**Where?**
Which area of the facility did the event occur?

**What?**
What type of equipment or instruments was involved in the event? Was anything wrong with the item?

What was the complaint or problem?

Was there any undesirable behavior involved?

What do you think led to the event?

## Interview form (cont.)

What other patients were being treated in the area?

What else was in progress in the area at the time?

What procedures, drawings, documents, or instructions were involved?  Was anything wrong with the item?

**Who?**

Which individuals were involved? What were their names and functions?

**How?**

How were items and personnel affected?

How did the event happen?

**How many?**

How many patients were affected?

How much of the unit was affected?

How many defects are known to exist?

How large are the defects?

Were other components or persons affected?

## Event and causal factor charting

### Overview

Event and causal factor (ECF) charting is used to assist the investigator in understanding the sequence of events and causes that led to the incident under investigation. Major events are not usually the result of single failures, but are the result of complex conditions that have evolved over a period of time and involve multiple work groups, systems, tasks/components.

ECF charting is very useful for evaluating complex events. It can be used to show the exact sequence of events from start to finish, including broken barriers, preexisting conditions, secondary events, inappropriate actions, and causal factors that produced and shaped the event.

ECF is an analytical technique or tool, it is not intended that the user become bogged down or overly burdened with the precise details of structuring and drawing the chart. Understanding and using the organizational and analytical concepts of the technique are more important.

- The ECF chart is a graphically displayed flow chart of an entire event. The heart of the ECF chart is the sequence of events and facts plotted on a time line.

- The beginning and ending points should be selected to capture all of the essential information pertinent to the situation.

- As the primary event line is established, additional situation features, such as related conditions, secondary events, and presumptions, should be added.

- Probable causal factors become evident as the chart is developed; often causal factors that were not obvious at the outset become evident through this technique.

- ECF charts are particularly useful for complex and complicated situations and are more meaningful than long narrative descriptions.

- The ECF chart provides an excellent opportunity to graphically display barriers, changes, cause and effect, and to show how they were involved in equipment and human performance situations.

## Event and causal factor charting (cont.)

It is important to understand the difference between how and why a situation occurs. The "how" in this case generally identifies the mechanism that created the situation (i.e. an equipment or human perform- ance condition, or a policy that drives the wrong behaviors.)

Why analyzes the reason the inappropriate action or condition occurred. For this reason, it is important to identify all the how's of a situation; otherwise some of the WHY's may be missed. Internal and external causal and situational information needed for the ECF chart can be obtained through interviewing along with and other analytical techniques, such as human error types/modes and organizational/programmatic failure modes

The cause-and-effect analysis of ECF charting identifies the cause(s), (i.e. the whys, for each of the primary effects or conditions.) In most situations determining a more detailed cause requires an iterative cause- and-effect process by treating the previous cause as an effect, (i.e. the adverse condition Y that cause an event Y is actually the result of another event X. ) The most precise cause applicable to the situation indi- cates where plant specific corrective actions are needed.

EFC charting is particularly good for situations involving equipment and human performance events in which the behavioral aspects are important. The technique can serve as a guide in directing the course of the evaluation and therefore it should be applied early in the task to obtain the most benefit. The chart is also very effective in illustrating the final report findings and conclusions. Corrective action(s) should be derived for each primary cause and for each secondary cause as warranted.

ECF charting contributes the following to an effective evaluation:

- Organizes situations and applicable data involved with the analysis.

- Shows the sequence of events from beginning to end. Presents the situation in a single glance (big picture).

- Stimulates development of other conditions, secondary events, presumptions, causal factors, changes, primary events, and control barriers.

## Event and causal factor charting (cont.)

- Incorporates results from other analyses. These results may expand the sequence of events, and provide more meaningful information.

- Provides cause-oriented explanations of the situation and inappropriate actions.

- Helps ensure objectivity.

- Provides a basis for beneficial changes to prevent future similar inappropriate actions.

### Practical application

The experience of many people participating in numerous accident/incident evaluations has led to the identification of six key elements in the practical application of ECF charting to achieve high-quality evaluations.

1. Begin early. As soon as the accumulation of factual information related to the event starts, begin construction of preliminary event sequence line with known primary events/happenings.

2. Proceed logically with available data. Events and cause factors usually do not emerge during the investigation in the sequential order in which they occurred. Initially, there will be many holes and deficiencies in the chart. Efforts to fill these holes and accurately track the event sequence and their contributing conditions will lead to deeper probing by evaluators and help uncover the true facts involved. In proceeding logically, it is usually easiest to use the last event as the starting point and reconstruct the pre-event and post event sequences from that vantage point.

3. Use an easily updated format—low charting software (i.e., Visio) or simply create by hand using Post-It Notes on a large sheet of paper. As the primary event line is established, additional situational features, such as related conditions, secondary events, barriers and presumptive conditions are added.

4. Gather facts using other evaluation techniques. Include the results of these techniques on the chart.

5. Develop conditions and causal factors to a greater detail. Include results of other evaluations techniques. Decide which actions are inappropriate.

6. Validate causes and conditions with results from other techniques.

## Event and causal factor charting (cont.)

### Definitions

- **Primary events**—actions or happenings directly leading up to or following the undesirable event. Events should be described with one subject and one verb, (i.e., "tubing ruptured" is an undesirable event v. "tubing has a crack" which describes a condition). Primary events are depicted as rectangles on the primary event line and are connected to each other by solid arrows.

- **Secondary events**—actions or happenings that impact the primary event , but are not directly involved in the undesired event. Secondary events are shown as rectangles below or above the primary event line and are connected to each other by arrows.

- **Terminal event**—the end point of the evaluation is shown as a circle at the end of the primary event line. This is usually the point that is being evaluated (e.g., medication misadministration, wrong surgical site, unanticipated outcome, etc.). The terminal event may appear at the middle of the chart to provide pre- and post event information.

- **Conditions**—circumstances that may have influenced the course of events and serve to provide additional details to the reviewer (e.g., vital signs, lab results, physician orders, etc.). Conditions are shown as ovals connected to each other or other events by lines.

- **Presumptive event**—action or happening that is assumed because it appears logical in the sequence, but cannot be proven. Presumptive events are shown as dotted rectangles.

- **Causal factor**—a factor that shaped the outcome of the situation. Causal factors are shown as ovals with the right end shaded. These are the root causes or contributing causes of the event.

- **Presumptive condition/causal condition**—a factor or condition that cannot be proven, but is assumed because it appears to logically affect another condition or event. Presumptive causal factors are shown as dotted ovals.

- **Primary effect**—an undesirable event or happening that was critical for the situation being evaluated to occur. Primary effects are shown as a diamond and are those events, which should not have occurred ( i.e. equipment failure, inappropriate action, etc.).

## Event and causal factor charting (cont.)

**Process**—(see figures included in this section)

a. Define the scope of the chart from initial information. Construct preliminary event line with known primary events. Each event must describe a single action or happening and should be precisely written using a short sentence containing one noun and one action verb. Each event should be derived logically from the one(s) preceding it and should be based on factual, valid information. Those that aren't derived logically should be enclosed in a dotted box or oval indicating it is an assumption. To construct the preliminary/primary event, take the following actions:

- Identify the beginning point.
- Identify the terminal event.
- Add other known primary events to develop a timeline for the event ("primary event line").

b. Evaluate initial information and documentation. Add known presumptive conditions to construct the preliminary event and causal factor chart.

c. Gather additional facts to complete the story or as questions arise from the chart construction. Develop the chart representations of conditions and causal factors to a greater detail.

- Identify those events which should not have occurred and were both inappropriate and essential to the development of the undesirable event (primary effects). Events should describe a single action or happening using a short sentence containing one noun and one active verb.

- Examine each primary effect and determine what conditions or causes allowed them to occur.

- For each condition identified, determine why that condition existed. Treat the condition as an effect and determine the cause for the effect. Identify conditions at the outset of the event, during the course of the event, and following the course of the event. Add these to the chart as ovals.

- Identify the factors causing or contributing to the outcome. Use cause and effect analysis to help identify relationships that exist around a primary effect to help identify contributing and root causes. Cause and effects analysis is based on the following principles:

## Event and causal factor charting (cont.)

- All undesirable events (i.e., equipment failures, human performance problems, etc.) are the effects of some cause (i.e. contributing cause or root cause)

- All undesirable events are caused to happen as a result of plant conditions, design, human performance, etc.

- For each condition (effect) identified, determine why it occurred (cause). The root cause(s) of an event can be determined by examining the cause and effect relationships that surround the primary effects (i.e., undesired event). For example, "the tubing had a crack" is a statement of a condition (effect), "why" the tubing had a crack would lead to the cause of the condition (cause, root cause).

- Physical/administrative barriers, which were broken, should be noted on the chart as broken bars.

- Ensure facts support conclusion.

d. Continue to investigate and develop the chart until one of the following limits is reached:

   •The cause is outside the control of the plant staff
      •The correction of the cause is determined to be cost prohibitive
      •The primary effect is fully explained
      •There are no other causes that explain the effect being evaluated

## Event and causal factor charting (cont.)

### TYPICAL SYMBOLS FOR EVENT AND CAUSAL FACTOR DIAGRAMS

1. Enclose all events (actions or happenings) in rectangles.

2. Enclose all conditions in ovals.

3. Connect primary events by solid arrows.

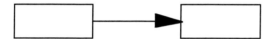

4. Connect secondary events with arrows.

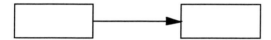

5. Connect conditions to other conditions and/or events using lines.

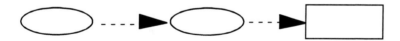

6. Presumptive events, causal factors, or conditions are shown by dotted rectangles or ovals.

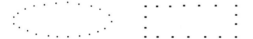

7. Terminal events are enclosed in a circle and can be placed at any point on the chart.

8. The primary sequence of events is depicted in a straight horizontal line with the primary events connected with arrows.

9. Relative time sequence is left to right.

---

## Event and causal factor charting (cont.)

10. Secondary event sequences, contributing causal factors, and causal factors are depicted above or below the primary event line.

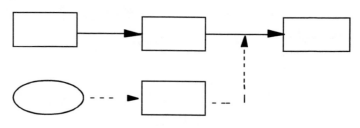

11. Barrier.    Failed Barrier

12. Change.

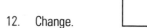

13. Primary effects are shown as diamonds.

14. Causal factors are shown as ovals which are shaded at one end.

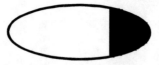

15. Terminal event is shown by a circle.

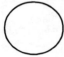

### EVENT AND CAUSAL FACTOR CHARTING PROCESS

Step 1—Construct preliminary event sequence line with known events. Identify initiating event, terminal event and any known primary effects (things that went wrong and caused the terminal event). Include how and when the event occurred and the consequences.

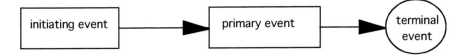

Step 2—Add secondary events, conditions and presumptive conditions to the preliminary event sequence line. Identify the condition that let up to the primary effect.

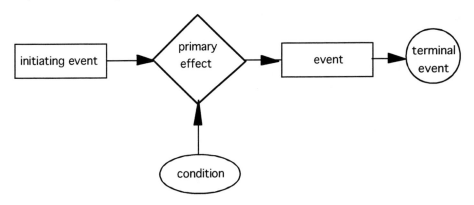

Step 3—Identify gaps and gather new facts from additional investigation.

Step 4—Integrate results form other analysis techniques (i.e. barrier analysis.)

Step 5—Add new information to the preliminary chart.

Change analysis

## Overview

Change analysis looks at events by analyzing differences between what was expected and what actually happened. It asks what differences have occurred to cause the event or activity to be different from previously successful performances.

Change analysis is a process that can be used to determine the contributing causal factors of events. The determination that contributing event factors are due to a change in some practice can lead the evaluators to better conclusions involving required corrective actions.

The fundamental process of change analysis involves the following six steps:

1. Situational determinations
2. Determination of similar, but event-free situations
3. Comparison of both situations
4. Recording of dissimilarities
5. Analysis of differences for impact on the event
6. Incorporating these differences into contributing causal factor.

Not recognizing a compound change (e.g., a change made five years previously, combined with a change made recently) or the introduction of a gradual change as compared with an immediate change is a potential shortcoming of change analysis.

### The basics

Change analysis is a process that can be used to determine the contributing causal factors of events. The determination that contributing event factors are due to a change in some practice can lead the investigator to better conclusions involving required corrective actions.

## Change analysis (cont.)

The fundamental process of change analysis involves the following six steps:

### 1. Situational determination

Evaluation of the situation surrounding the event is critical to the change analysis process. Emphasis should be placed upon determining all possible contributors to the event. These include: time of event, personnel, equipment, procedures, physical surroundings, event severity, etc.

### 2. Similar, but event-free event determination

Evaluate similar situations where a problem or event did not occur. If possible, choose a situation where the majority of contributors are the same.

### 3. Comparison of both situations

Compare the event situation with the nonevent situation. Look for dissimilarities in event and non-event contributors. Be careful to consider all differences no matter how insignificant that they may appear.

### 4. Write down all differences

Dissimilarities between the event and nonevent situations should be written down. It is preferable to group differences under major contributing categories. Refer to situational determination for examples.

### 5. Analyze the differences for effect on the event

Differences between the event may be as obvious as the time of day or as nebulous as the same instructions being given by a different person. Each difference must be individually dissected for its impact on the event.

### 6. Incorporate contributing differences into the event causal factors

Contributing differences are caused by a change in some practice. The investigator must determine what mechanism created this change. Once identified, this change must be altered or eliminated to prevent recurrence.

## Change analysis (cont.)

**Change analysis questions:**

**Why now, not before?**

Consider the following:

- Time of day
- Day of week
- Season
- Year

- Holiday
- Overtime
- Other

**Why here, not there?**

Consider the following factors:

- Physical location
- Step in the process
- Work group
- Facility
- Field v. lab or office location

**Other change analysis effects?**

████████████████  **Barrier analysis**  ████████████████

## Overview

A Barrier analysis is a systematic method used to identify possible root causes and contributing factors. For this purpose, "barrier" is defined as an administrative or physical control that is designed to prevent or inhibit an undesirable action from reaching its' victim. Barriers are established to ensure consistent and desired behavior by equipment and plant personnel. A single barrier is rarely relied upon in high-risk operations. Generally, barriers are diverse and numerous, (i.e.. in the defense-in-depth concept).

In general there are three specific modes of barrier failure

1. The barrier fails to provide the protection envisioned.
2. The barrier was not in place at the time of the event.
3. The barrier was knowingly or unknowingly circumvented.

Barrier analysis is helpful in pinpointing subtle contributing factors as it examines each of the connections in a failure path scenario. In using this method, each link is viewed as a barrier to the failure and the following questions should be asked:

- Why does the barrier not break the link?

- If there is no existing barrier, is a barrier required?

- If there are existing barriers but they did not work, ascertain the factors that make up each barrier and determine why they were ineffective.

While barrier analysis identifies missing or defective barriers, it has one weakness. If the investigator does not recognize all of the failed barriers, the analysis may be incomplete. For this reason, when the investigator is unable to determine the root cause, due to perceived time pressures, the tendency is to jump to lack of barriers as the root cause and recommend adding more procedures and review to ensure that the particular event will never happen again. This quick fix often results in burdensome processes, which can cause more problems. Therefore it is recommended that barrier analysis be used in conjunction with other techniques or methods.

## Barrier analysis (cont.)

**Details**

In general barrier analysis deals with a target and a threat: The threat is prevented from reaching the target by a barrier. Typically the process requires establishing the target, identifying the threat to the target, and then determining what barriers can or should be in place to prevent the threat from causing an event, (i.e,. what will prevent the threat from reaching the target).

When an evaluation is begun, evaluators should think in terms of barriers. Established barriers may vary and analysis of them is dependent on the knowledge of the reviewer. Regardless of variations in barriers, cause analysis provides the framework for barrier assessment because it focuses on precise barrier categories that have proven to be keys to equipment and human performance problems. Corrective actions from cause evaluation usually include the addition or modification of control barriers.

Barriers can take many forms and may include one or more of the following:

**1. Physical barriers**
- Engineered safety features
- Safety and relief devices
- Human factored designs
- Redundant equipment
- Locked doors
- Electrical shields (protection devices)
- Radiation shielding
- Monitor alarms and reminders

**2. Organizational and program control barriers**
- Inservice and training
- Supervision
- Patient safety improvement programs
- Lessons learned programs

**3. Program monitoring barriers**
- Peer review

**Barrier analysis (cont.)**

- Common cause analysis
- Self-assessments

## 4. Administrative barriers
- Standards of case
- Practice guidelines
- Policies and management practices
- Training and education
- Licenses and certifications
- Qualification tests

## Barrier analysis considerations

- Identify failed barriers that allowed the event to progress. This evaluation usually occurs early in the investigation and continues until completion.

- Determine how the barrier failed, (e.g., patient safety alert process barrier failed because it was not used).

- Determine why the barrier failed,(e.g., process was not used because the lab technician felt the problem would be fixed soon and would not result in a need to use it).

- Validate the results of the analysis with information learned from documentation and interviews.

The following questions are intended to assist in determining what barriers may have failed.

- Were there any barriers that did not perform their functions?  Why?
- Did the barriers mitigate or increase the severity of the event?  Why?
- Were any physical barriers not functioning as designed? Why?
- Was the barrier design adequate?  Why?
- Were the barriers adequately maintained?
- Were the barriers inspected prior to use (if applicable)?

**Barrier analysis (cont.)**

- Is the affected process/system designed to withstand the conditions/situation without the barriers in place? Why?
- What changes in process or practice could have prevented the unwanted condition? Why?
- What human response could have prevented the unwanted condition? Why?
- What equipment could have prevented the unwanted condition? Why?
- What other controls are the barriers subject to? Why?
- Was this event foreseen by anyone?
- Is it possible to have foreseen the event? Why?
- Is it practical to have taken further steps to reduce the risk of the event occurring?
- Can this reasoning be extended to other similar systems/processes?
- Were adequate human factors considered in the design of the environment, equipment, and process?
- What additional human factors could be added? Should be added?
- Is the system/process user friendly?
- Is the system/equipment adequately labeled for ease of operation?
- Is there sufficient technical information for operating equipment properly? How do you know?
- Is there sufficient technical information for maintaining the equipment properly? How do you know?
- Is the problem instruction or procedure related?
- What information is necessary to correctly perform the task?
- How was information presented to users?
- Did users have enough information to be reasonably expected to perform the task properly?
- Did the environment mitigate or increase the severity of the event? Why?
- What could have been done to prevent the event, disregarding all economic considerations?
- What would you have done differently to have prevented the event, considering all economic concerns?

## Barrier analysis worksheet—health care example

| Consequences | Barriers that should have precluded the event | Barriers assessments (why the barriers failed) | Corrective action recommendations |
|---|---|---|---|
| | | | |
| | | | |
| | | | |
| | | | |
| | | | |
| | | | |
| | | | |
| | | | |
| | | | |

## Overview

Task analysis is a tool that can be used on virtually any event evaluation; during cause determination it focuses on the steps to be performed and how they are performed. It is reasonable to assume one of the first priorities when beginning an evaluation is to determine as much as possible about the task(s) and actions associated with the event or condition. This will require a review of documents that describe the assigned task or procedure (checklists, turnover logs, clinical instructions, etc.) in an effort to determine what the task was about, how it was to be performed, and the desired effect on the equipment. This process is called a task analysis and may be done in two ways: paper and pencil task analysis or the walk-through task analysis. Frequently, parts of both will be performed.

### Paper and pencil Task Analysis

Paper and pencil task Analysis is a method of task analysis where a task is broken down on paper into sub-tasks identifying the sequence of steps, actions, instructions, tools, equipment associated with performance of a particular task.

Objectives:

- Break down the task into different sub-tasks, actions, or steps that are expected to be performed during the relevant activity.

- Identify information, controls and displays, instruments, medications, materials and other requirements for the performance of the task.

- Identify potential questions (concerning deficiencies in practice or technique, procedures, controls/displays and training, etc.) to be asked when interviewing the individuals involved.

- Establish a general understanding of how the task being evaluated is to be performed.

- Identify potential problems with the performance of the task such as inadequate instructions, procedures, inappropriate working or environmental conditions, etc.

**Task analysis (cont.)**

Steps in paper and pencil task analysis:

1. Obtain preliminary information so you know what the person was doing when the problem or inappropriate action occurred.
2. Focus on the part of the procedure or task of interest.
3. Obtain necessary background information.
   - Relevant checklists or procedure(s).
   - Inservice instruction, etc.
   - Interview personnel who have performed the task—but not those who will be observed—to obtain understanding of how the task should be performed.

4. Divide the task of interest into individual actions or steps.
5. Write step name or action in order of occurrence on the task analysis worksheet.

## Paper and Pencil Task Analysis Worksheet

| Steps | Who | Required action | Instruction or job aid I | Instrument or tools | Remarks/questions |
|-------|-----|-----------------|--------------------------|---------------------|-------------------|
|       |     |                 |                          |                     |                   |
|       |     |                 |                          |                     |                   |
|       |     |                 |                          |                     |                   |
|       |     |                 |                          |                     |                   |
|       |     |                 |                          |                     |                   |
|       |     |                 |                          |                     |                   |
|       |     |                 |                          |                     |                   |
|       |     |                 |                          |                     |                   |
|       |     |                 |                          |                     |                   |
|       |     |                 |                          |                     |                   |

## Walk-through task analysis

A walk-through task analysis is a method in which personnel conduct a step-by-step reenactment of their actions for the observer without carrying out the actual function. If appropriate, it may be possible to simulate performing the task rather than conducting a walk-through.

### Objectives
- Determine how a task was really performed.
- Identify problems in human factors design, discrepancies between procedural steps and what is actually done, training, etc.

### Preconditions
- Participants should be the people who have previously performed the task successfully.

### Steps in cause-and-effect task analysis

1. Obtain preliminary information so you know what the person was doing when the problem or inappropriate action occurred.

2. Decide on task of interest.

3. Obtain necessary background information.
   - Relevant procedure(s).
   - Procedures, practice guides, literature, inservice packages, etc.
   - Interview personnel who have performed the task—but not those who will be observed—to obtain understanding of how the task should be performed.

4. Produce a guide outlining how the task will be carried out, indicating steps in performing the task and key controls and displays so that:

   - You will know what to look for.
   - You will be able to record actions more easily.

## Task analysis (cont.)

- A procedure with key items underlined is the easiest way of doing this.
- The best guide is a completed task analysis worksheet (refer to paper and pencil task analysis).

5. Thoroughly familiarize yourself with the guideline/instruction and decide exactly what information you are going to record and how you will record it.. Consider the following:

- You simply may want to check off each step it occurs.
- Discrepancies and problems may be noted in the margin or in a space provided for comments, adjacent to the step.

6. Select personnel who normally perform the task. If the task is performed by a group, all members should play the same role they fulfill when carrying out the task normally.

7. Observe personnel walking through task and record their actions and use of displays and controls. Note discrepancies and problem areas.

- Walk-through task analysis is normally used to recreate a situation that had human performance problems in a way that provides a sense of how the event occurred.

- Conducting the task under the conditions, as nearly as possible, that existed when the event occurred will provide the best understanding of the event causal factors.

- Walk-through analysis may be done in slow motion, stopping the task if there are question.

- Walk-through analysis may be done in real time to better identify time-related problems.

8. Summarize and consolidate any problem areas noted. Identify probable contributors to the event.

## Instructions for performing stream analysis:

1. Using the information collected from the multiple events being reviewed, create **one "sticky note" for each of the inappropriate actions** identified. (Using 2" x 2" sticky notes works best.) At the top of the sticky note, write the keyword(s) that will help you identify the "gist" of the inappropriate action represented by the note. Leave space at the bottom of the sticky note for the key word of the associated sub-group (from the next step). You may have more than 20 sticky notes as a result of this step. That's OK!

2. Based on the total population of inappropriate actions you've identified, develop a list of sub-groups that represent the 4–5 major themes of organizational/programmatic weakness represented by the group (e.g., knowledge weaknesses, lack of guidance, lack of supervision, failure to self-check, etc.).

3. Now, sort the sticky notes into the 4–5 major sub-groups, based on their stated symptoms and correlation to one of the organizational or programmatic concepts you identified. Write the sub-group assigned to each issue at the bottom of its' sticky note as a reminder of your selection. (You may shuffle these notes issues around multiple times so you'll need to remember what "group" it came from.) *If possible, use a computer program (i.e. Visio or Power Point) to perform the remaining steps.*

4. Develop a chart to depict the different streams, or sub-groups of weaknesses you identified in step #2 above. At the top of the chart, place one box across the sheet (horizontally) for each of the sub-groups identified in step #2 above. (Refer to the top figure on the next page.) Make sure this chart is large enough to allow you to place all the sticky notes on it at one time and draw linkages between the issues. By the time you have "coded" all the sticky notes representing various inappropriate actions and mistakes, and placed them in groups on your chart it should look like the bottom figure on the next page.

## Example stream analysis chart

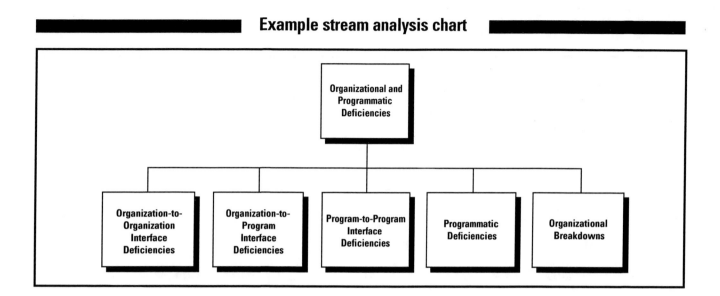

## Example stream analysis chart

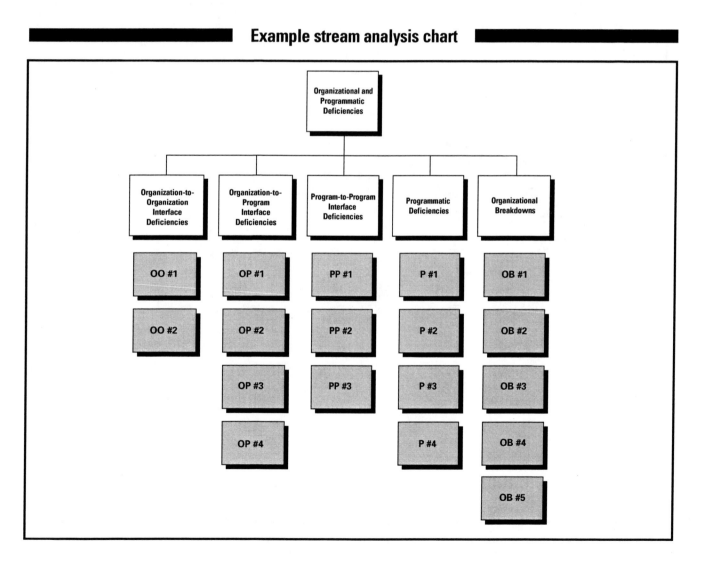

## Stream analysis (cont.)

5. Identify interconnections between causes and effects for each of the issues identified on the sticky notes by asking some simple cause and effect questions based on information gleaned from the investigation. For each of the notes ask: "Is there another sticky note (inappropriate action) on this chart that appears to drive this issue?" Where your answer is yes; draw a line from the sticky note containing the driving (causal) factor to the note containing the receiving (effects) factor. (Place only one arrowhead per line, pointing at the receiving factor.) (Refer to the figure below )

## O&P stream analysis diagnostic chart

**Stream analysis (cont.)**

Boxes with arrows going into them are symptoms. Boxes that have only outgoing arrows are causes. The cause(s) are now the focus of your investigation.

6. Once you have finished the cause and effect annotation for each inappropriate action, do the following:

   a. Highlight the cause box(es) (those that only have arrows coming out of them).

   b. Step back and analyze the chart to identify core problems, stories and themes associated with the causes you've identified. Annotate them with different colored highlighters or markers. (Don't worry if there is more than one theme or story associated with your chart. There may be as many as five or six.)

   c. Simplify the chart by removing any uninvolved sticky notes. But keep them close by as your continued investigation may reveal a yet unidentified linkage.

   d. Jot down a summary of each of the causes and "themes" identified in the stream analysis.

   e. Assign the causal themes to a team member for validation and verification.

7. Have team members investigate their assigned "themes" by looking for supporting or refuting evidence within the data and information collected during the investigation. Once they have completed the review of information and themes, annotate those that are supported by information and details found in the analysis. Also annotate those that are refuted by the existence of information contained in the analysis, explaining what information refutes their identification as a cause in this analysis.

8. Document root cause(s) driving multiple issue themes and develop a story (a paragraph or two) that describes each. Benchmark with others (in and outside your organization) to determine the most viable actions to correct the cause(s) and prevent recurrence.

9. Develop corrective actions to address the causal themes.

10. Develop an effectiveness review plan to evaluate the impact of corrective actions after implementation.

In general, stream analysis can be used successfully by experienced personnel to evaluate most situations. Nevertheless, stream analysis (one type of organizational and programmatic root cause analysis) is most effective when accomplished by individuals with specialized training in the common cause analysis techniques. These advanced cause analysis techniques and analytical methods allow investigators to apply numerical values to each block of the stream analysis so that a calculation sequence is produced that represents individual and accumulative failure rates. However, training and experience in this area are required as the numerical values are based on industry data and then refined by the evaluator to fit the particular circumstances evidenced in the causal themes.

**The benefits of stream analysis include the following:**

- It provides a structured process that facilitates a common understanding of fundamental core issues.

- It results in a greater commitment for what needs to be done due to the weight of the multiple events included in the collective analysis.

- It provides a visual tool for communication of issues to stakeholders and line managers.

- It is a simple, yet flexible approach that can be used on large data sets with any level of detail.

- It provides a structured process that facilitates a common understanding of fundamental core issues.

- It results in a greater commitment for what needs to be done due to the weight of the multiple events included in the collective analysis.

- It provides a visual tool for communication of issues to stakeholders and line managers.

- It is a simple, yet flexible approach that can be used on large data sets with any level of detail.

## Selection and comparison of root cause analysis techniques

| Method | Usage | Advantages | Disadvantages |
|---|---|---|---|
| Event and causal factor charting | • Develops a story line<br>• Good for all events<br>• Helps report writing | • Provides a graphical display of the event<br>• Incorporates results of other techniques<br>• The most flexible technique | • Can be time consuming<br>• Can be confusing for novices |
| Barrier analysis | • Procedure or admin. problems.<br>• Human performance<br>• Identifies physical and admin barriers and reviews them for effectiveness.<br>• Determines the "why's". | • Helps identify causal factors and corrective actions.<br>• Good addition to the event and causal factors chart. | • Danger of not recognizing all failed barriers. |
| Change analysis | • Single problems.<br>• Investigating equipment problems.<br>• Useful when you do not know where to start.<br>• When the causes of actions are unclear or when change is suspected. | • Simple, quick, good where there is a record of successes to compare.<br>• Generates questions for interviews.<br>• Supplements event and causal factor charting. | • May generate more questions than it answers.<br>• Gradual or compound changes can be overlooked.<br>• Danger of incorrectly defining the change. |
| Task analysis | • To become familiar with the task, how it is done.<br>• To break a task into subtasks.<br>• To identify conditions in training and procedures. | • Helps identify where deviations are made from the approved method.<br>• Helps identify questions and improvement areas for further investigation. | • Only tells what was supposed to happen.<br>• Time consuming.<br>• Most effective when performed by personnel responsible for the task. |

## Work environment factors (conditions inducing human error)

| People | Tasks | Arrangement | Environment |
|---|---|---|---|
| Leadership | Planning | Work area | Lighting |
| Morale | Coordination | Seating | Noise |
| Communication | Workload | Layout | Climate |
| | Multi-tasking | | Activity |

## Human factors (conditions inducing human error)

| | | | |
|---|---|---|---|
| Input and output | Human capability | Arrangement | Environment |
| Visual display | Text/graphics symbols/codes | Workspace layout | Light |
| Auditory display | Anthropometry | Component layout | Noise |
| Controls | Tools and devices | | Climate |
| | Human control | | Motion |
| | Physical work | | |

Suggested Reading:
Sanders & McCormick *"Human Factors in Engineering and Design."*

# Human error / inappropriate action failure mode chart

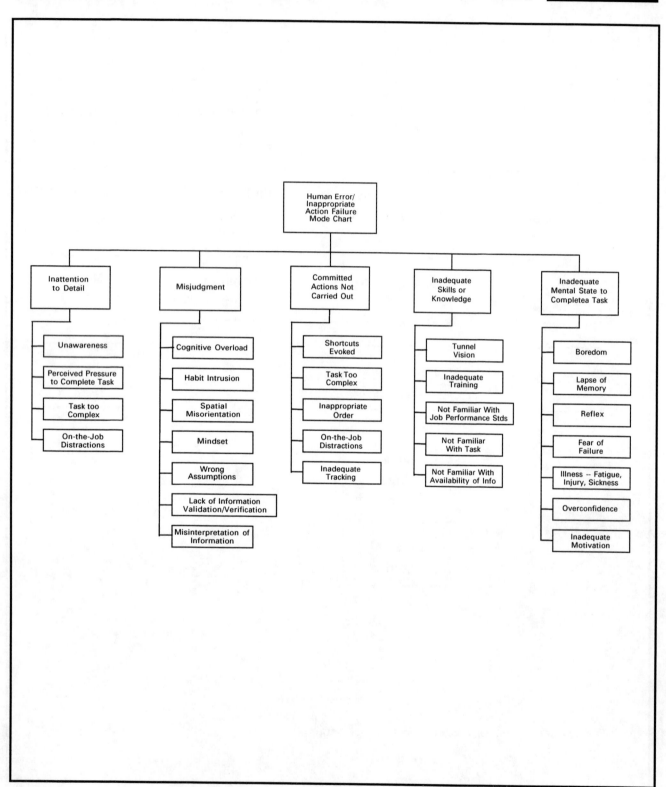

# Organizational and programmatic diagnostic chart

```
                        ┌─────────────────────┐
                        │    Organizational   │
                        │   and Programmatic  │
                        │   Diagnostic Chart  │
                        └─────────────────────┘
```

| Organization-to-Organization Interface Failures | Organization-to-Program Interface Failures | Program-to Program Interface Failures | Programmatic Deficiencies | Organizational Breakdowns |
|---|---|---|---|---|
| Inadequate Interface Among Organizations | Lack of Commitment to Program Implementation | Lack of Interface Requirements | Insufficient Programmatic Detail | Inadequate Organizational Structure |
| Excessive or Lack of Overlap in Functions | Lack of Program Monitoring or Management | Conflicting Program Requirements | Inadequate Scope | Lack of Attention to Emerging Issues |
| | Lack of a Program Evaluation Process | Inadequate Interface Requirements | Excessive Implementation Requirements | Inadequate Work Prioritization |
| | Lack of Organizational Authority for Program Implementation | | Inadequate Self-Verification Process | Inadequate Communication Within The Organization |
| | | | | Inadequate Job Skills, Work Practice, or Decision Making |

## Executive management failure mode chart

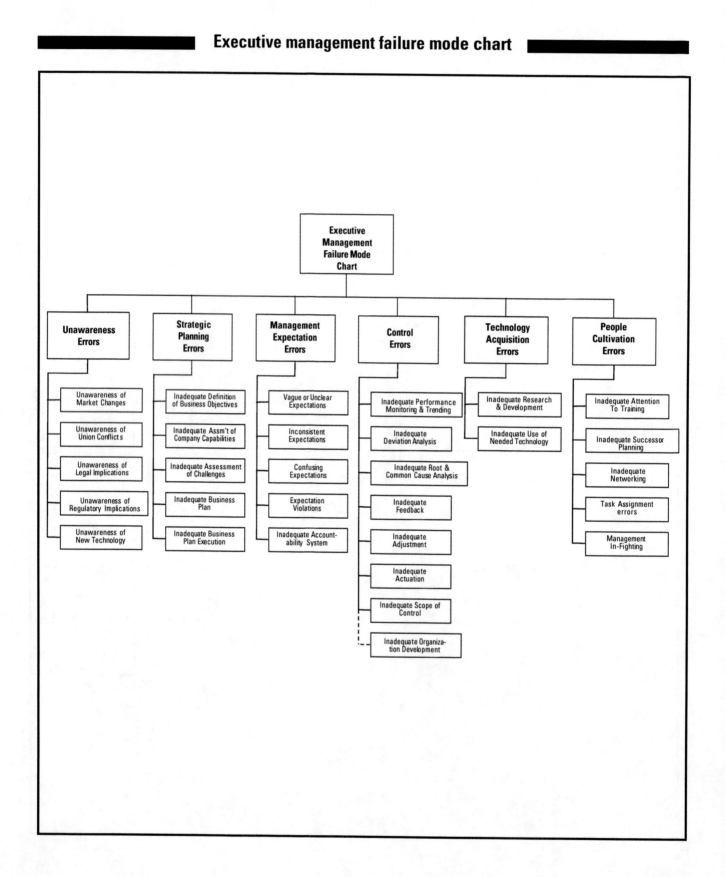

## The top 12 high-risk behaviors causing sentinel events in health care

1. Caregivers communicate without using clarification questions and repeat-backs.

2. Caregivers leave patients unattended without providing the patient the ability to get help.

3. Caregivers do not document the patient medical record, in an adequate or timely manner.

4. Patients don't promptly report unexpected pain, discomfort, or changes to their caregivers.

5. Physicians do not formally communicate with patients and other caregivers prior to surgical or other critical activities.

6. Caregivers do not consult with other experts when unexpected outcomes occur.

7. Physicians do not fully explore or communicate the risk of treatment, risk-factors, or adverse drug side effects.

8. Caregivers administer treatment or dispense medications without verifying the "5Rs": Right patient, right medication, right dose, right time, right route.

9. Caregivers use equipment or perform tasks when they are inexperienced or when it has been a relatively long time since they last performed the task.

10. Patients receive or take medication without verifying it against the original prescription.

11. Caregivers are noncompliant with established rules, regulations or requirements or patients are noncompliant with caregiver instructions.

12. Caregivers provide care when they are not "fit-for-duty", (e.g., fatigued or under the influence of alcohol or drugs).

## The top 12 high-risk situations causing sentinel events in health care

1. Changes to treatments or medications are not explained to the other caregivers or patient.

2. Caregivers are distracted immediately before or during the administration of treatments or medications.

3. Shortage of caregivers or adequate equipment to care for the patient.

4. Patient condition is not adequately monitored following critical activities or significant changes in treatments.

5. Poorly trained or inexperienced caregivers, who are unsupervised or under-supervised, are allowed to perform critical tasks.

6. High-alert drugs or "look-alike/sound-alike" drugs are used in treatment without verification.

7. Multiple procedures are conducted during a single activity, e.g. surgical operation.

8. Multiple physicians are involved in the care of a single patient.

9. Patients are under restraint without close observation.

10. Patients are incapacitated or physically impaired without close observation.

11. Uncontrolled, unproven, unchecked, or modified equipment is used for drug administration or other treatment interventions.

12. Medical care is provided under a human error prone situation (e.g. dark room, noisy setting, shift turnover, etc.) without appropriate compensatory actions.

*Source: Performance Improvement International, based on approximately 91% of the 360 sentinel events studied.*

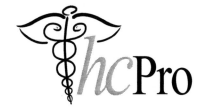

# Related Products from HCPro

## Books

### Failure Modes and Effects Analysis: Building Safety into Everyday Practice

The JCAHO's patient safety standard requires hospitals to conduct at least one FMEA per year to identify and improve high-risk failure modes. However, hospitals continue to struggle with the practicality of turning FMEA theory into practice. This book moves beyond theory and

- provides an in-depth look on how to properly conduct an FMEA—with practical examples and advice from real-life FMEAs
- Walks you, step-by-step, through the FMEA process
- Includes hands-on tools, best-practice advice, and discussion of potential pitfalls to avoid
- Offers case studies on the most problematic, high-risk areas

### Performance Improvement: Winning Strategies for Quality and JCAHO Compliance, Third Edition—Plus CD/ROM

This is the third edition of our award-winning compliance tool! The book and companion CD/ROM have just been updated to reflect the significant changes in the JCAHO's survey process. The JCAHO has revamped its PI standards—specifically around ORYX, FMEA, and core measures—and made PI one of the only remaining planned interviews in the 2004 survey process. You need to know how to respond to the changes to comply! Plus—in addition to keeping PI and quality of care a main focus of its survey process, the JCAHO is adding patient safety as a critical area as well. This book includes a new chapter on patient safety in response to the JCAHO's increased focus on this crucial area, and an educational PowerPoint presentation on CD/ROM.

### JCAHO 2003 and 2004 National Patient Safety Goals: Successful Strategies for Compliance

Hospitals continue to struggle to meet the intent of the JCAHO's National Patient Safety Goals. This step-by-step tool breaks down each of the requirements within the JCAHO's seven National Patient Safety Goals and provides you with a series of best-practice tips that you can easily implement. You'll receive

- CASE STUDIES from hospitals across the country that are successfully complying with these seven Goals

- sample POLICIES, including patient identification and verification of operative site policies
- step-by-step ADVICE, such as how to prevent wrong-site/ patient/procedure surgery
- sample FORMS and CHECKLISTS, including a surgery verification checklist

### Preparing Your Patient Safety Program for JCAHO Survey

Your patient safety program initiatives have never been under more scrutiny than right now. From the JCAHO's new Patient Safety Goals to new survey expectations, you need to make sure your patient safety program is up to par. This book provides you with

- plain-English EXPLANATIONS of the JCAHO's 2004 patient safety standards and step-by-step ADVICE on how to comply with them
- sample CHECKLISTS, FORMS, and DOCUMENTS
- INSIGHT into how your patient safety initiatives will be surveyed
- TIPS and GUIDANCE on implementing a patient safety program, failure modes and effects analysis (FMEA), sentinel events, and root cause analysis
- EXAMPLES of the types of patient safety questions surveyors might ask staff

## Newsletters

### Briefings on JCAHO

This 12-page monthly newsletter is the respected voice of authority for practical, independent guidance on succeeding in the accreditation process at thousands of hospitals nationwide. It will keep you up to speed on all JCAHO changes and provide invaluable insight into how the new JCAHO survey process unfolds. Whether readers are new to the survey game or seasoned professionals, each newsletter offers quick reading "how-to" advice on meeting the JCAHO standards. You'll receive tips and information from accreditation experts that would otherwise cost you dearly in consulting fees and research!

### Briefings on Patient Safety

From medication management to the Patient Safety Goals, there has never been more focus on your facility's patient safety initiatives than right now. This monthly resource was created exclusively to help you provide a safe environment of care for your patients. From best-practice information regarding medication management to ensuring that your patient safety program stands up to JCAHO scrutiny, you'll have the tools you need to succeed!

---

**To obtain additional information, to order any of the above products, or to comment on** *Maximizing Patient Safety with Advanced Root Cause Analysis* **please contact us at:**

**Mail:**
HCPro
P.O. Box 1168
Marblehead, MA 01945

**Toll-free telephone:** 800/650-6787
**Toll-free fax:** 800/639-8511
**E-mail:** *customerservice@hcpro.com*
**Internet:** *www.hcmarketplace.com*

---